Emergency Triage

This book is dedicated in the loving memory of our dear friend and colleague Professor Janet Marsden.

Writing the 4th edition was nowhere near the fun experience of our previous versions due to the simple fact Janet was not here with us. What we sorely missed this time round was her sharp intellect and commonsense approach to problem solving, not to mention her unique sense of humour that would lighten the toughest of days.

Despite Janet not sitting with us to discuss charts or write chapters, she continues to leave her mark on every page. Her ideas and words remain woven throughout this book and that truth brings a warm smile as we acknowledge, honour and remember our beloved and much missed friend.

Emergency Triage

Manchester Triage Group

FOURTH EDITION

EDITED BY

Jill Windle

Kevin Mackway-Jones

Stephanie Allmark

Janet Marsden

Advanced Life Support Group

A charity dedicated to saving life by providing training

WILEY

This edition first published 2027

Edition History
BMJ Publishing Group (1e, 1996); Blackwell Publishing Ltd (2e, 2005); John Wiley & Sons, Ltd (3e, 2013)

Registered Offices
John Wiley & Sons, Inc., 111 River Street, Hoboken, NJ 07030, USA
John Wiley & Sons Ltd, New Era House, 8 Oldlands Way, Bognor Regis, West Sussex, PO22 9NQ, UK

For details of our global editorial offices, customer services, and more information about Wiley products visit us at www.wiley.com.

The manufacturer's authorized representative according to the EU General Product Safety Regulation is Wiley-VCH GmbH, Boschstr. 12, 69469 Weinheim, Germany, e-mail: Product_Safety@wiley.com.

Wiley also publishes its books in a variety of electronic formats and by print-on-demand. Some content that appears in standard print versions of this book may not be available in other formats.

Library of Congress Cataloging-in-Publication Data applied for:

Paperback ISBN: 9781394266654

Cover Design: Wiley

Image Credits
Timer image © George Dolgikh / Adobe Stock
Pearl image © AllebaziB / Adobe Stock

Set in 10/12 Montserrat by Straive, Pondicherry, India
Printed and bound by CPI Group (UK) Ltd, Croydon, CR0 4YY
C9781394266654_270826

Contents

Editors

Jill Windle, Triage Consultant Nurse, Advanced Life Support Group. Retired Lecturer Practitioner in Emergency Nursing, Salford Royal Hospitals NHS Foundation Trust and University of Salford

Kevin Mackway-Jones, Retired Consultant Emergency Physician, Manchester Royal Infirmary and Manchester Children's Hospital; Medical Director, North West Ambulance Service

Stephanie Allmark, Paramedic with North West Ambulance Service, Emergency Department Nurse and Clinical Development for the Manchester Triage Group

Janet Marsden (1961–2018), Professor of Ophthalmology and Emergency Care and Director, Centre for Effective Emergency Care, Manchester Metropolitan University

Members of the original Manchester Triage Group

Kassim Ali, Consultant in Emergency Medicine
Simon Brown, Senior Emergency Nurse
Helen Fiveash, Senior Emergency Nurse
Julie Flaherty, Senior Paediatric Emergency Nurse
Stephanie Gibson, Senior Emergency Nurse
Chris Lloyd, Senior Emergency Nurse
Kevin Mackway-Jones, Consultant in Emergency Medicine
Janet Marsden, Senior Ophthalmic Emergency Nurse
Sue McLaughlin, Senior Paediatric Emergency Nurse
Rosemary Morton, Consultant in Emergency Medicine
Karen Orry, Senior Emergency Nurse
Barbara Phillips, Consultant in Paediatric Emergency Medicine
Phil Randall, Consultant in Emergency Medicine
Joanne Royle, Senior Emergency Nurse
Brendan Ryan, Consultant in Emergency Medicine
Ian Sammy, Consultant in Emergency Medicine
Steve Southworth, Consultant in Emergency Medicine
Debbie Stevenson, Senior Emergency Nurse
Claire Summers, Consultant in Emergency Medicine
Jill Windle, Lecturer Practitioner in Emergency Nursing

International Reference Group

Australia
Thomas Njoroge
Clare Toms
Catherine Wright

Austria
Andreas Lueger
Stefan Kovacevic
Willibald Pateter

Azores
Filipe Ribeiro

Brazil
Welfane Cordeiro
Maria do Carmo Paixã Rausch
Paula Tassia Barbosa Rocha

Canada
Brad Parlongo
Kathleen Pascuzzo

Chile
Leonardo Cabrera

Czech Republic
Jakub Dedek
Michal Pisar
Ondrej Rennet

Germany
Joerg Krey
Jochen Thiele
Ina Trzebiatowski

Italy
Gabriele Magnarell
Norbert Pfeifer
Elia Toccolini

Mexico
Noe Arellano Hernandez
Jesica Bravo
Elizabeth Hernandez Delgadillo

Netherlands
Joanne Blom
Nadine Jongmans
Roy Vanleen

New Zealand
Blair Andrews
Nic Toms

Norway
Stine Engebretsen
Germar Schneider

Poland
Bartosz Krasiński
Flis Krzysztof
Piotr Rychlik

Portugal
Paulo Freitas
Antonio Marques
Angela Valenca

Slovakia
Timea Uchaľová
Silvia Štefaníková

Slovenia
Majda Cotič Anderle
Vida Bračko
Renata Rajapakse

Spain
Gema Garcia Riestra
Richard Houghton
Josep Tortosa Ferrer

Switzerland
David Ertman
Maria Kundert
Nicole Theiler

UK
Stephanie Allmark
Kevin Mackway-Jones
Jill Windle

Preface to the fourth edition

It is amazing that it is 30 years since the core text supporting the Manchester Triage System, now generally known as the MTS, was first published. It feels like yesterday that the senior clinicians leading the local delivery of emergency medicine in what were accident and emergency departments in Greater Manchester were having weekly meetings during which they crafted the MTS as our local solution to our local problem. Since then, the MTS has been adopted by many urgent and emergency care systems around the world. It has also been joined by the very successful Manchester Telephone Triage and Advice (TTA) system that was derived as a support to the first book and is based on the same principles.

Fundamentally the system has not drastically changed since the first edition, which is testament to the vision, rigour and thousands of person hours poured into that first iteration. The fourth edition of *Emergency Triage* offers a complete rewrite of all the chapters, with detailed advice on how to successfully implement and sustain the MTS. At times it may read more like a manual than a reference book with the inclusion of case studies to enhance understanding, clearly setting out the 'how to use MTS in practice'. The charts are not dramatically different, there is one new chart, and the major incident charts are abandoned. The biggest change comes with the reordering of discriminators into a strict hierarchy, that flows through all charts and level of priority, to strengthen decision making by selection of the highest order discriminator each time the system is used.

By far the biggest change to the MTS, since the original publication, comes from a new approach to the triage of patients in acute mental health crisis. This change is based on a focused Delphi study that included experts from six stakeholder groups and was designed to encourage parity of esteem between patients with mental health and physical health presentations. The results have been operationalised by incorporating 19 new discriminators into the existing presentation flow charts.

Perhaps the most significant changes are invisible to the clinical triage practitioner. These involve the governance structures that have been put in place to standardise the international decision-making processes, and a re-energised effort to continuously assess and improve quality. Our role as editors of this book and as members of the Manchester Triage Executive Board, that ultimately makes the decisions regarding content, is to make sure the tool is usable, accurately represents best clinical practice and supports the delivery of good inter- and intra-user reproducibility. Your role as triage practitioners using this tool is to use it correctly. Outcomes of triage that result from using the tool incorrectly are not MTS errors, but rather errors of triage delivery. Training and continuous quality measurement and improvement are key to this standard being upheld.

We sincerely hope you enjoy the rest of this book and find much in it that can develop your practice.

Kevin Mackway-Jones, Jill Windle and Stephanie Allmark
Manchester, 2026

Preface to the first edition

Every day, emergency departments are faced with a large number of patients suffering from a wide range of problems. The workload varies from day to day and from hour to hour and depends on the number of patients attending and what is wrong with them. It is absolutely essential that there is a system in place to ensure that these patients are seen in order of clinical need, rather than in order of attendance.

In the past year great steps have been made towards establishing a National Triage Scale in the United Kingdom; this follows on from similar work in Australia and Canada. This book is intended to allow practitioners of triage to work to a set standard when applying national scales to the patients presenting to their departments. The members of the multi-professional consensus group that designed this methodology hope that individual practitioners will use it to inform the triage process and ensure that their decisions are both valid and reproducible.

This manual contains the basic knowledge necessary for triage practitioners to begin to build their competence in performing triage. It is hoped that practitioners will find a useful source reference and *aide-memoire*.

Kevin Mackway-Jones, 1996

CHAPTER **1**

Introduction and background

How it all began

There is a prelude to the development of the Manchester Triage System (MTS) that has never been acknowledged or documented and as this fourth edition is published, and 30 years of MTS celebrated, it is only right and proper the full story be told.

In 1993, Jill Windle and Kevin Mackway-Jones worked together in the Accident and Emergency (A&E) Department at Stockport Infirmary, Manchester. The previous year the UK government had published 'The Patient's Charter', an initiative to raise standards within the NHS. Included in this national standard was the waiting time for an initial assessment in A&E, which stated 'patients would be seen immediately and their need for treatment assessed'. Sitting in the coffee room, Jill shared her frustration with Kevin as to how an initiative that was supposed to raise standards, had become little more than a 'Hello nurse'. The initial assessment was reduced to merely a quick glance at patients to meet the time-sensitive target of an initial assessment within 5 minutes of arrival. She discussed her ideas to develop a more robust triage system, one that could be taught to all nurses. The objective was that no matter who was making the assessment, the decision making would be safe and reproducible; despite the new standard, triage was still intermittent, with no consistency in prioritisation. During these discussions Kevin began to sketch out a rough algorithm on the back of a napkin, with just four priorities at this stage. They quickly realised if they could further develop these charts all patients would have a standard assessment, aiding the triage nurses to assign a priority.

During the next few months, a small working party of senior nurses and doctors at Stockport Infirmary developed and implemented a robust triage system rather than merely replacing triage with an initial assessment. The triage nurse's role was detailed and for the first time became a designated role allocated per shift.

Initially, five algorithms were developed and implemented:

- Immediate (life threat)
- Conscious level
- Limbs
- Wounds
- Eye

As can be seen from Figure 1.1, the first 'discriminators' were formed, although they were not titled as such during this phase.

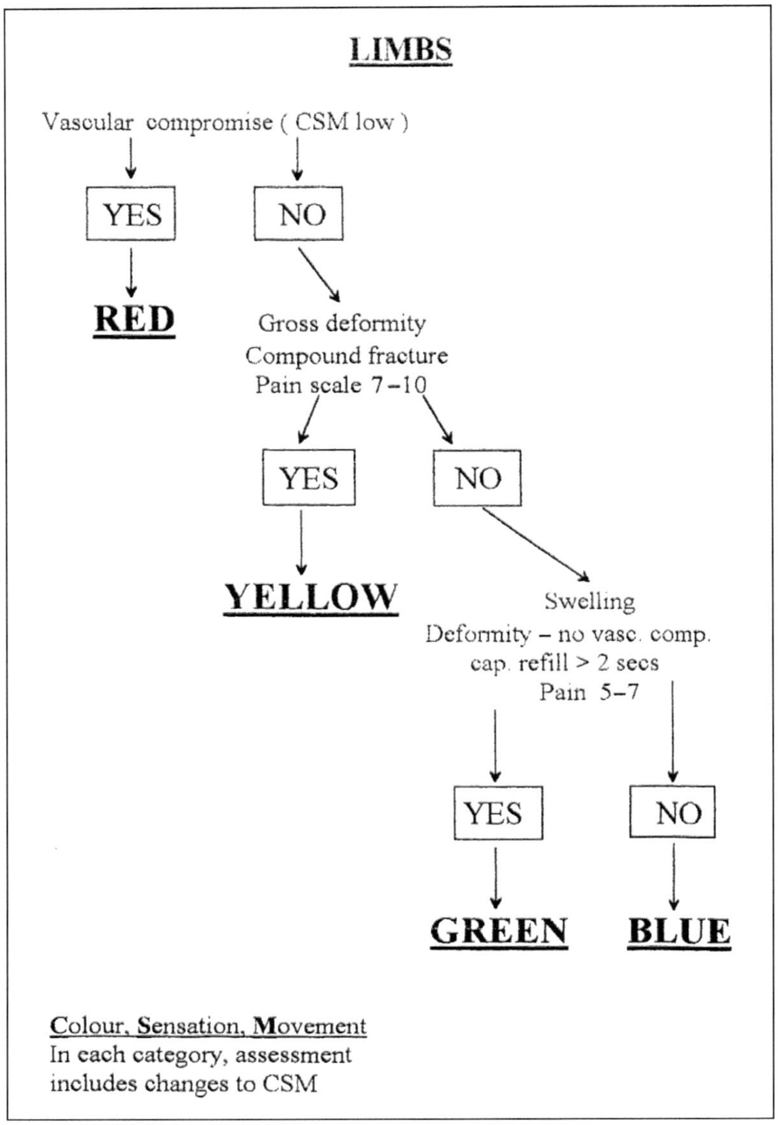

Figure 1.1 Limbs algorithm

Alongside the first charts, other developments included:

- Documentation to quickly and accurately record the triage event
- Pain assessment added as a key component
- A training programme devised and rolled out
- Audit established, with many of the original criteria still in use today
- Patient satisfaction surveys conducted

This impromptu discussion during a coffee break would become the basic premise of the Manchester Triage System.

Background and overview

Triage is one of the most important clinical risk management tools. Employed in urgent and emergency care worldwide, triage is used to safely manage patient flow when clinical need exceeds capacity. Triage systems are intended to ensure care is defined according to patient need, not departmental management, and that it is delivered in a timely manner by trained triage practitioners.

Early emergency department triage was intuitive rather than methodological, and was therefore neither reproducible between practitioners nor auditable. The Manchester Triage Group was first set up in November 1994 with one notable member being Professor Janet Marsden. The aim of the group was to establish consensus amongst senior emergency nurses and emergency physicians about triage standards. It soon became apparent that the group's aims could be set out under five headings that required development:

- Common nomenclature
- Common definitions
- A robust triage methodology
- A training programme
- An audit guide

Nomenclature and definitions

A review of the sparse triage nomenclature and definitions in use at the time revealed considerable differences across emergency departments, but despite this variation, it was apparent there were common themes running through the different triage systems.

Collating commonalities, the group agreed on a new common nomenclature and definition system. Each of the five categories, now referred to as priorities, was given a number, a colour and a name and was defined in terms of ideal maximum time to first contact with the treating clinician. At meetings between representatives of emergency nursing and emergency medicine nationally, this work informed the derivation of the UK triage scale shown in Figure 1.2.

Number	Colour	Name	Timeframe
First	Red	Immediate	0 minutes
Second	Orange	Very urgent	10 minutes
Third	Yellow	Urgent	60 minutes
Fourth	Green	Standard	2 hours
Fifth	Blue	Non-urgent	4 hours

Figure 1.2 UK triage scale

As practice has developed over the past 30 years, five-part triage scales have been established around the world and acknowledged as the gold standard. The target times themselves are locally set, being influenced by politics as much as by medicine, particularly at lower priorities, but the concept of varying clinical priority remains current.

Triage methodology

In broad terms, triage methods vary in their focus, with any of the following being predominant:

- Diagnosis
- Resource allocation
- Disposal
- Clinical priority

The Manchester Triage Group quickly decided that this triage methodology would be designed to allocate a clinical priority – a decision based on three major tenets. First, the aim of the triage encounter is to aid clinical management of the individual patient, which is best achieved by accurate allocation of a clinical priority. Second, the length of the triage encounter is such that any attempts to accurately diagnose a patient are doomed to fail, as this activity requires a consultation rather than a rapid and focused triage assessment. Finally, it is apparent that diagnosis is not accurately linked to clinical priority. Priority reflects several aspects of the patient's presentation, not just the diagnosis; for example, patients with a final diagnosis of ankle sprain can present with severe, moderate, mild or no pain, and their clinical priority will differ to reflect this finding.

In outline, the MTS requires practitioners to select from a range of patient presentations, then starting at the highest priority to seek a limited number of signs and symptoms as they move down each level. The signs and symptoms that discriminate between the clinical priorities are termed *discriminators* and they are set out in the form of algorithms known as *presentation flowcharts*. Discriminators that indicate higher levels of priority are sought first, and to a large degree patients who are allocated to the standard/4/green clinical priority are selected by default (see Chapter 2).

Priority and management

It is easy to become confused between the clinical priority and the clinical management of a patient. Priority requires enough information being gathered to enable the patient to be placed into one of the five defined triage priorities. Management often requires a much deeper understanding of the patient's needs, and may be affected by many extraneous factors such as time of day, the state of staffing and number of beds available. Furthermore, the availability of services for patients will fundamentally affect individual patient flow. Separately staffed 'streams' of care for particular patient groups will run at different rates but this must not alter underlying clinical priority which affects the order of care within, rather than between, streams in such a system.

Triage in practice

The fourth edition of *Emergency Triage* offers detailed advice on how to successfully implement and sustain the MTS. At times it may read more like a manual than a reference book, with the inclusion of case studies to enhance understanding and clearly setting out the 'how to use MTS in practice'.

This book, in conjunction with the accompanying Manchester Triage System Provider Course, provides the baseline knowledge, confidence and competence necessary to facilitate the introduction of a standard triage method. The process has been highly successful, not only in the UK where the system originated, but across the world where many countries, seeking a standard for triage in their healthcare systems, have implemented the MTS. Reading this book and attending a course will not produce instant expertise in triage – rather, this process will introduce the method and allow practitioners to develop confidence in using MTS as a first step towards competence (see Chapter 3). Once initial training and subsequent supervision of practice is completed it must be followed up by regular audit of individual triage practitioners and evaluation of their use of the system.

Beyond triage in the emergency department

The MTS was originally designed specifically for emergency departments but has proved over time to be applicable in numerous settings. Across a range of clinical areas, for example medical, surgical or paediatric assessment units, the system is implemented in exactly the same way as in an emergency department and as such provides all the benefits of a robust triage system.

Many users of the MTS have recognised that the outcome of selecting a presentation flowchart and reaching a priority has further utility when used to direct patients to a particular part of the service. The chart selection/priority assignment process results in the placement of individual patients into one of the 54 charts across five priorities, essentially providing 266 slots or possible streams. These designations can be used to drive pathways of care in systems that have taken to 'streaming' by developing a presentation priority matrix. Particular presentation–priority combinations, for example wounds–green or chest pain–orange, may be appropriate to designated streams, in this instance minor injuries and resuscitation room, respectively (see Chapter 5).

Triage audit

The original triage group spent considerable time trying to pin down 'sentinel diagnoses'; that is, a diagnosis that could be identified retrospectively and used as a marker of accurate triage. However, it became apparent that even retrospective diagnosis could not accurately predict actual clinical priority at presentation.

Successful introduction of a robust audit method is essential to the future of any standard methodology since reproducibility between individual practitioners and departments must be shown to exist (see Chapter 7).

Worldwide use of MTS and International Reference Groups

The MTS is recognised throughout the world as a gold standard for triage. The spread of MTS across the globe has been truly remarkable as an ever-increasing number of countries seek a triage system that is both safe and reproducible. With a conservative estimate of over 150 million patients triaged using MTS worldwide per year (and rising), it is undoubtedly the most widely used triage system in the world.

Governance of the MTS is a fundamental part of the work of the Manchester Triage Group Executive Board, based within the Advanced Life Support Group (ALSG), a registered charity dedicated to saving lives by providing training. The Manchester Triage Group support the many teams of clinicians who introduce and maintain MTS in their designated countries. These groups, known as International Reference Groups (IRGs), abide by a set of roles and responsibilities and are an integral part of the MTS family. In return the IRGs contribute to the ongoing development of the system, the body of evidence and the exemplary patient safety record that MTS upholds.

Triage pearls

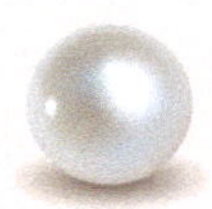

When this symbol appears within the chapters it denotes a sharing of facts about MTS and tried and tested methods to improve the use of the system in practice. These 'triage pearls' are taken from the training programme and often provide useful insights and examples that aid understanding of the system. Also, the triage pearls set the record straight, busting the various myths and misunderstandings about MTS that circulate and are unhelpful to triage practitioners.

Summary

Triage is a fundamental part of clinical risk management in all settings where clinical load exceeds clinical availability. Emergency triage promulgates a system that delivers a teachable, auditable method of assigning clinical priority within urgent and emergency care settings. It is not designed to judge whether patients are appropriately in the correct setting, but to ensure that those who need care receive it. The MTS has been shown to have functions beyond the initial concept of prioritisation when used to monitor patients and signpost to streams of care determined by local provision and actual availability.

For the most up to date information on the Manchester Triage System visit the triage website at **www.triagenet.net**.

CHAPTER **2**

The triage method and decision-making process

Introduction

The method that underpins the Manchester Triage System (MTS) is designed to ensure the triage practitioner rapidly assigns a clinical priority to each patient. The system selects patients with the highest priority first without making any assumptions about the diagnosis. Emergency departments and urgent care facilities are largely driven by the patients' presenting signs and symptoms and the lack of focus on diagnosis is, therefore, deliberate.

Five-step process to triage decision making

1. Identify the problem
2. Gather and analyse information related to the solution
3. Evaluate all the alternatives and select one for implementation
4. Implement the selected alternative
5. Monitor the implementation and evaluate outcome

Identifying the problem

Clinical practice is geared around the concept of the patient's *presenting complaint*, that is the main sign or symptom identified by the patient or carer.

The list of MTS presentation flowcharts (Box 2.1) covers almost all presentations to urgent and emergency care for both adults and children. The list, charts and contents were initially compiled following considerable discussion and testing and have been subsequently refined, in both this and previous editions. Changes made to the presentation flowcharts are based on changes in practice, current evidence base and international consultation. The presentations fall broadly into the categories of illness, injury, children and abnormal and unusual behaviour relating to mental health. In the case of children, paediatric-specific charts are only developed when there is differing physiological or developmental signs or symptoms and are established by evidence-based studies (see Further reading). In most other instances the charts are applicable to both adults and children.

The first part of the triage method requires the practitioner to select the most appropriate presentation flowchart from the list.

Each chart contains a series of discriminators that allow the clinical priority to be determined.

A key feature of the method is that the charts are consistent in their approach, since it is recognised that the presenting complaints of a few patients may initially indicate that more than one presentation flowchart could apply. However, only one chart should be used and a detailed

Box 2.1 The 54 presentation flowcharts

Manchester Triage System
Emergency Triage 4e Presentation Flowcharts

Emergency Triage

- Abdominal pain in adults
- Abdominal pain in children
- Abscesses and local infections
- Abuse and neglect
- Allergy
- Apparently drunk
- Assault
- Asthma
- Back pain
- Behaving strangely
- Bites and stings
- Burns and scalds
- Chemical exposure
- Chest pain
- Collapse
- Crying baby
- Dental problems
- Diabetes
- Diarrhoea and vomiting in adults
- Diarrhoea and vomiting in children
- Ear problems
- Eye problems
- Facial problems
- Falls
- Fits
- Foreign body
- GI bleeding
- Head injury
- Headache
- Irritable child
- Limb problems
- Limping child
- Major trauma
- Mental illness
- Neck pain
- Overdose and poisoning
- Palpitations
- Pregnancy
- PV bleeding
- Rashes
- Self-harm
- Sexually acquired infection
- Shortness of breath in adults
- Shortness of breath in children
- Sore throat
- Testicular pain
- Torso injury
- Unwell adult
- Unwell baby up to 12 months
- Unwell child
- Unwell newborn up to 28 days
- Urinary problems
- Worried parent
- Wounds

understanding of how to choose the most specific chart, related to the patient, is essential for the accurate use of emergency triage.

To aid understanding, the following example of a case offers a simple illustration of the accurate chart selection process:

> **Example case**
>
> A 46-year-old man presents to triage with a 2-day history of feeling generally unwell. Today he has started with a severe headache and has some stiffness in his neck.

The case example may initially lead the triage practitioner to use the unwell adult chart but further scrutiny of what the patient is saying should lead to the selection of a more specific chart such as headache, which is his main complaint. The patient also mentions he has a stiff neck, therefore the neck pain flowchart could be used and, as many of the discriminators in these two charts are consistent, the patient would be triaged at the same priority and the same discriminator selected.

Gathering and analysing information

The patient's presentation will largely dictate which of the presentation flowcharts is selected (Figure 2.1).

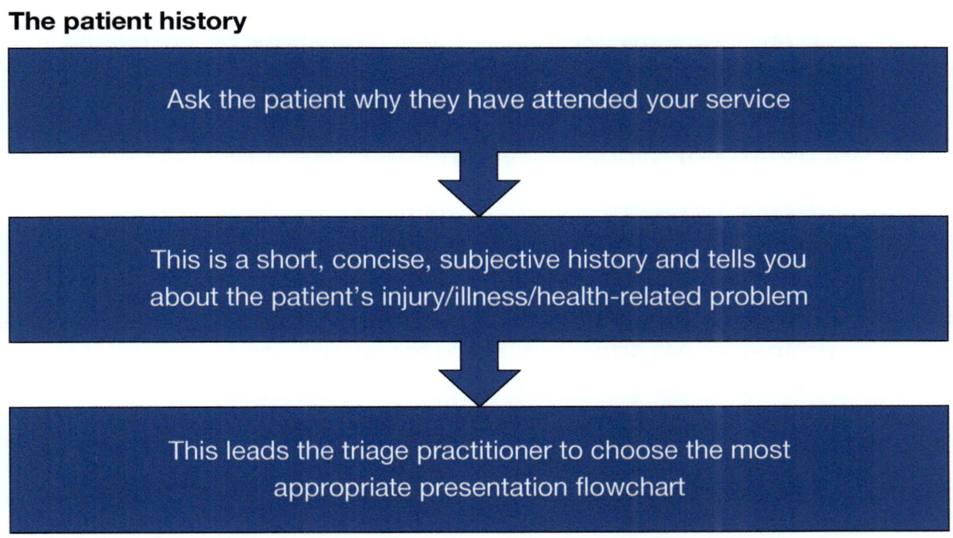

Figure 2.1 The patient history

Following the most specific chart selection, information must be gathered and analysed to allow the actual priority to be determined. The MTS uses a reductionist methodology, the triage practitioner always begins at the top of the chart, in the highest priority, and works down the list of discriminators to find the information required. The presentation flowchart structures this process by showing key discriminators at each level of priority. In reality there could be many discriminators that pertain to the patient's presentation, but the selection of only one discriminator is required, and this would be the first highest order discriminator at which the answer posed by the discriminator question is positive. Discriminators are deliberately posed as questions by the triage practitioner to facilitate the triage assessment.

General and specific discriminators

Discriminators, as their name implies, are factors that discriminate between patients, such that they allow them to be allocated to one of the five clinical priorities. The discriminators are termed general or specific and are arranged in strict hierarchical order. As well as the airway, breathing, circulation and disability (ABCD) hierarchy, that has always existed in priority 1 (red), this edition sees a detailed hierarchy within each of the priorities. Table 2.1 illustrates the hierarchy and the rationale behind this consistent ordering of discriminators.

Table 2.1 Strict hierarchy of discriminators

Airway	General and specific discriminators related to airway
Breathing	General and specific discriminators related to breathing
Circulation	General and specific discriminators related to circulation
Disability	General and specific discriminators related to disability / consciousness
Environment	Mainly temperature-related discriminators
Signs	Current signs and symptoms we ask about using relevant clinical questioning
Behaviour	Incorporates mental health and any behavior-related discriminators
History	Those things we ask about or clarify related to the history of the presentation
Pain	Specific discriminators, such as a site of pain, appear first and in alphabetical order followed by the general discriminators
Recent issues	Anything within the last 7 days that prevents the patient moving into the blue priority

Translated versions will use the UK alphabetical order to make sure the charts are identical for all triage practitioners, no matter where they are practicing.

General discriminators

General discriminators are quite simply the backbone of the MTS and provide the framework around which the specific discriminators are arranged. There are six groups of general discriminators; these discriminators are a recurring feature of the charts and apply to all patients irrespective of their presentation. They appear time and again throughout the charts, and a detailed comprehension of all the general discriminators is essential to an understanding of this triage method.

The six sets of general discriminators also appear in the same hierarchical order within each of the presentation flowcharts they apply to.

1. Life threat
2. Conscious level
3. Haemorrhage
4. Temperature
5. Pain
6. Acuteness

Life threat

To a practicing emergency nurse or emergency physician life threat is perhaps the most obvious group of general discriminators. Broadly speaking, this group of general discriminators recognises that any cessation or threat to the vital airway, breathing and circulation (ABC) functions places the patient in priority 1 (red).

Patients who are unable to maintain their own airway for any length of time have an insecure airway. Absence of breathing is defined as no respiration or respiratory effort as assessed by looking, listening and feeling. Inadequacy is a more difficult concept but, in general, patients who are failing to breathe well enough to maintain adequate oxygenation have inadequate breathing. There may be an increased work of breathing, signs of inadequate breathing or exhaustion. Absence of pulses is only diagnosed after palpation over a central pulse for 5 seconds. Shock can be more difficult to identify but the classic signs include sweating, pallor, tachycardia, hypotension and reduced conscious level (Figure 2.2).

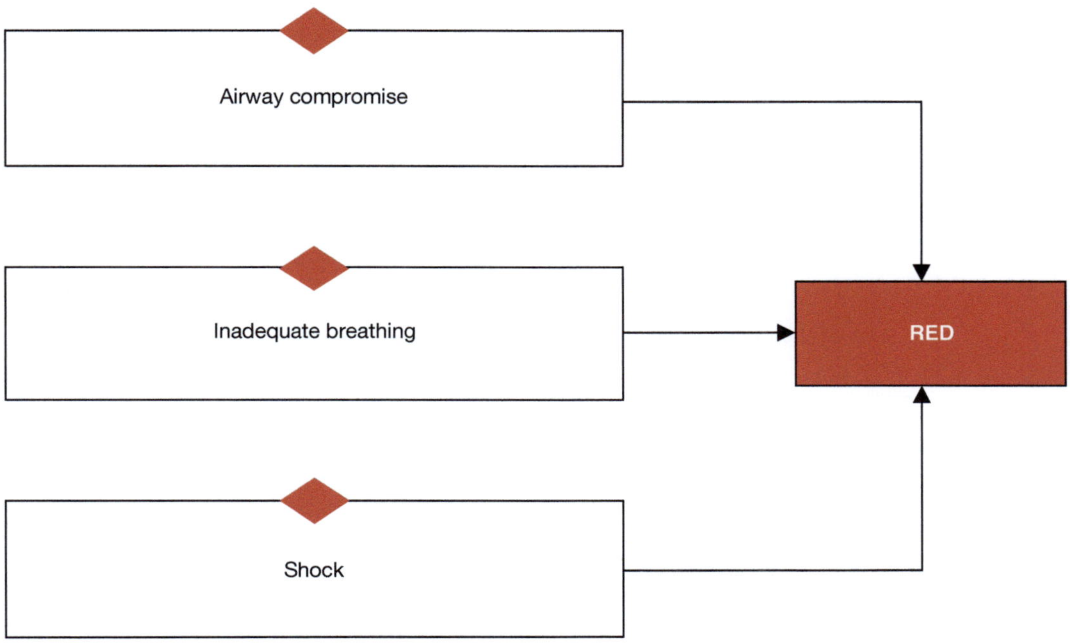

Figure 2.2 Life threat

Conscious level

Conscious level is considered differently for adults (Figure 2.3) and children (Figure 2.4). In adults, only currently fitting patients are always triaged as priority 1 (red), while *all* unresponsive children are placed in this clinical priority. Adult patients with altered conscious level (responding to voice or pain only or unresponsive) are triaged as priority 2 (orange), as are children who respond to voice or pain only. All patients who are now alert but have a history of unconsciousness should be triaged as priority 3 (yellow).

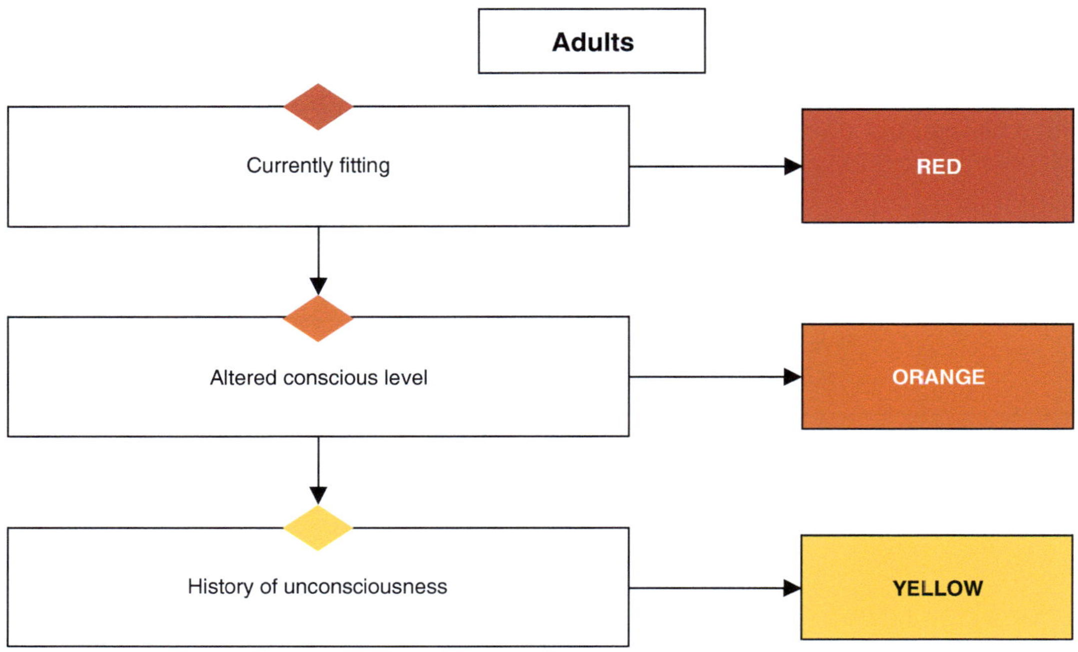

Figure 2.3 Conscious level in adults

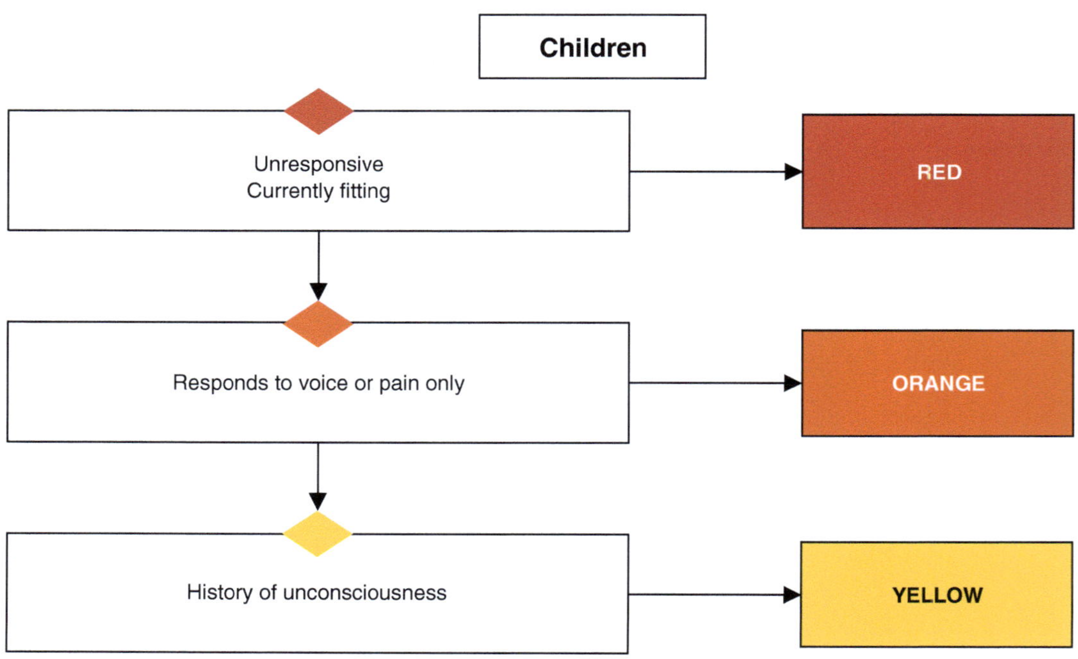

Figure 2.4 Conscious level in children

The fact that all patients with alterations in conscious level are allocated to the very urgent priority may be at odds with current practice; this is especially so regarding the clinical priority given to patients who are intoxicated or under the influence of drugs. Two points need to be made about this patient presentation. Firstly, the aetiology of alterations in level of consciousness is largely irrelevant in determining the risk to the patient, as an altered conscious level due to drugs or alcohol is clinically as important as an altered conscious level due to other causes. Secondly, most intoxicated patients do not have an altered level of consciousness. Specific points about the allocation of clinical priority to patients who are apparently drunk are dealt with in the presentation flowchart of that name.

Haemorrhage

Haemorrhage is a feature of many presentations, particularly, but not exclusively, those involving trauma. The haemorrhage discriminators are exsanguinating, uncontrolled major or uncontrolled minor (Figure 2.5). The use of how successful attempts to control the haemorrhage are is deliberate since continuing bleeding has a higher clinical priority. In practice it can be difficult to decide which category a particular haemorrhage falls into; the definitions of the discriminators are designed to help the practitioner make this decision. Exsanguinating haemorrhage is present if death will ensue rapidly unless bleeding is stopped. A haemorrhage that is not rapidly controlled by the application of sustained direct pressure, and in which blood continues to flow heavily or quickly soaks through dressings, is described as an uncontrollable major haemorrhage, while that in which blood continues to flow slightly or ooze, is described as uncontrollable minor haemorrhage.

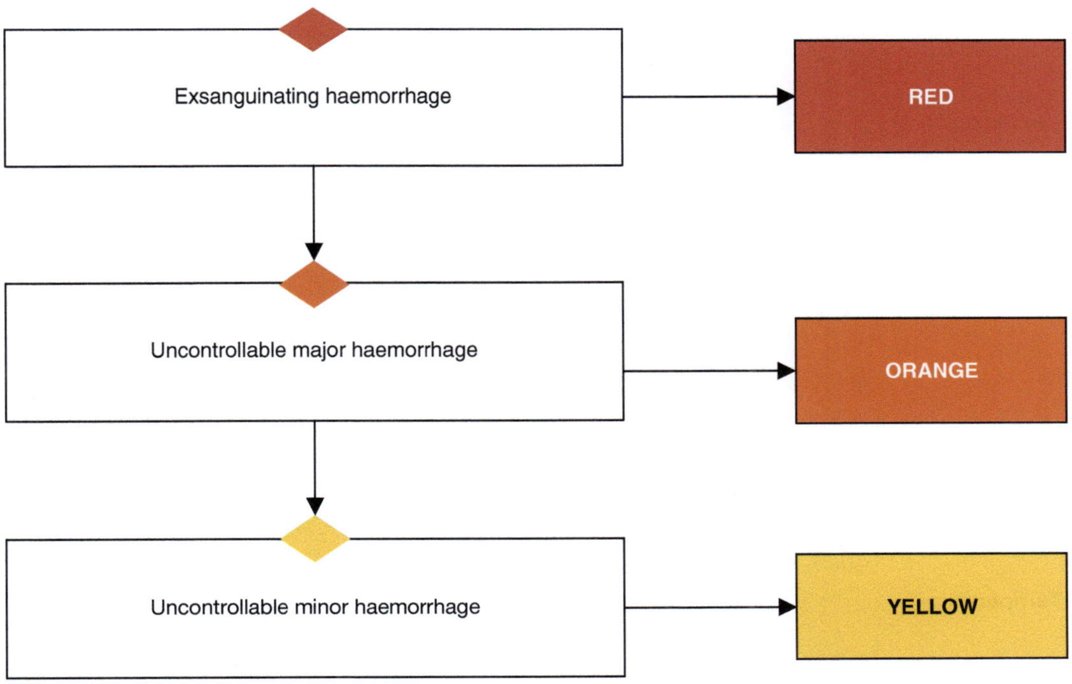

Figure 2.5 Haemorrhage

Temperature

Temperature is used as a general discriminator and accurate measurement of the temperature should be a part of the triage process where indicated within a chart. Clinical impression of skin temperature is also important and crucial where immediate assessment of core temperature is not possible.

If the skin feels very hot, the patient (if over 12 months of age) is said to be clinically very hot and would correspond to a temperature of 41°C or above. Similarly, if the skin feels hot, the patient is clinically said to be hot and this corresponds to a temperature of 38.5–40.9°C. A patient with warm skin fulfils the discriminator of warmth and this would indicate a temperature of 37.5–38.4°C.

Patients with cold skin can be said to be clinically cold; a core temperature of 35°C or less matches this general discriminator.

Important temperature differences are built into the system to recognise babies, with immature immune systems, who require a higher priority (see Further reading). The hot baby (from birth to 12 months) will always be triaged as priority 2 (orange). For all patients over the age of 12 months, the following discriminators in the temperature group apply (Figure 2.6): a very hot patient (1 year and above) will always be triaged as priority 2 (orange), while a hot patient will be triaged as priority 3 (yellow) and a warm patient priority 4 (green). Patients who are cold, irrespective of age, will be allocated to priority 2 (orange).

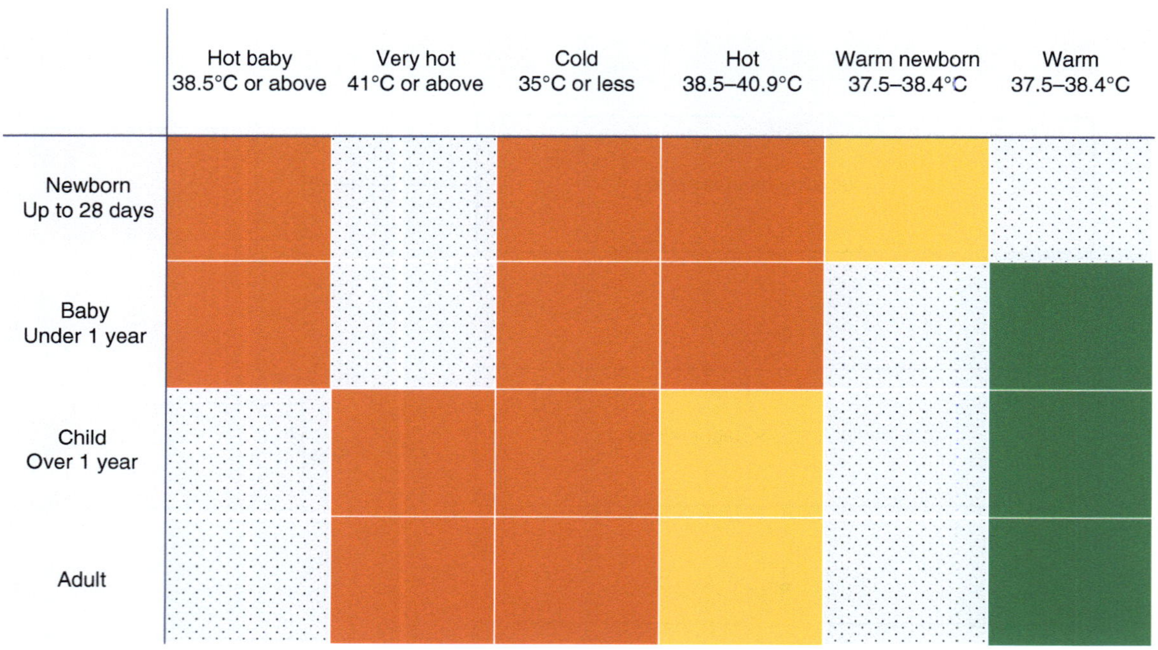

Figure 2.6 Temperature

Pain

From the patient's perspective, pain is a major factor in determining priority. The use of pain as a general discriminator throughout the presentation flowcharts recognises this fact and implies that every triage assessment should include an assessment of pain (Figure 2.7). Pain assessment is dealt with in Chapter 4 and readers are referred there for a detailed discussion.

In general terms, the discriminator severe pain is intended to imply pain that is unbearable, often described as the worst ever, while moderate pain refers to pain that is bearable but intense. Any patient with a lesser degree of recent mild pain should, if no other discriminators suggest a higher triage category, be allocated to priority 4 (green) and not to the non-urgent priority 5 (blue).

The general pain discriminators describe the intensity or severity of pain only. Other characteristics of pain, such as site, radiation and periodicity, may feature as specific discriminators in particular presentation flowcharts.

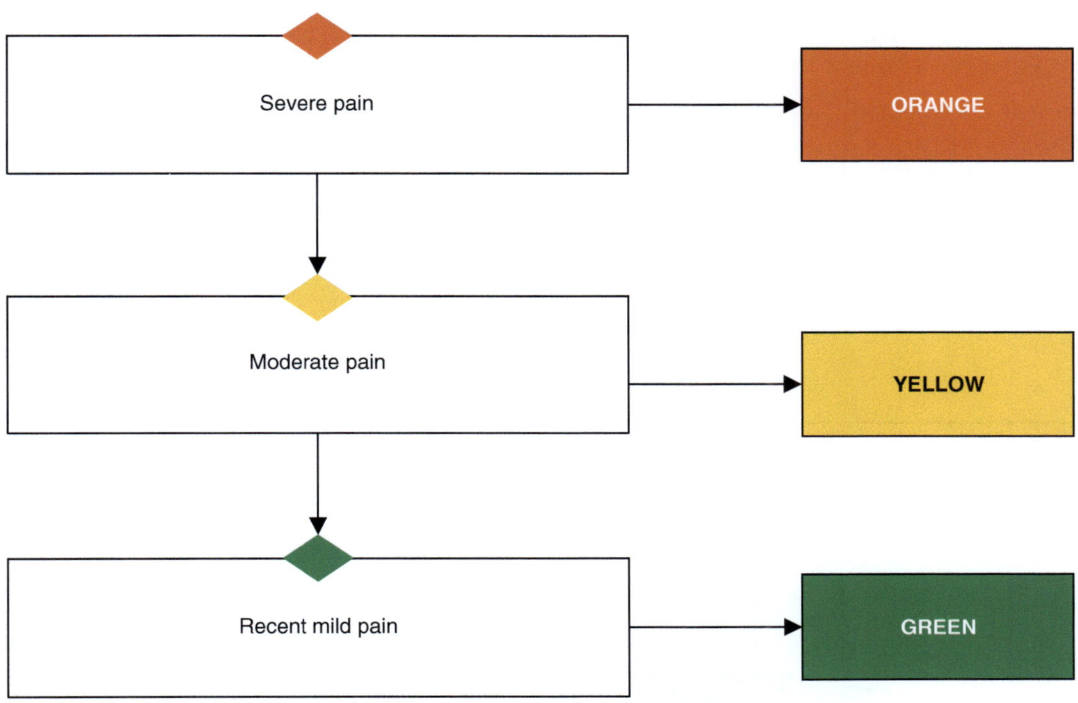

Figure 2.7 Pain

Acuteness

Within the triage method certain conventions have been used to help with consistency. The term 'abrupt' is used to indicate onset within seconds or minutes and 'acute' indicates a time period within 24 hours. Recent signs and symptoms are those that have appeared within the past 7 days.

Whilst most clinicians have no problem accepting that the acuteness of onset can help indicate the clinical priority, it is slightly more controversial to argue that chronicity, in this case greater than 7 days, is used to define a non-urgent problem. However, on reflection, it is intuitive that the relatively long time that the problem has been present indicates that the patient can be allocated the non-urgent priority without clinical risk as *'none of the above discriminators apply'* in the hierarchy of these charts. The triage method is such that the presence of any other discriminator, be that general or specific, relevant to the patient presentation will have resulted in the allocation of a higher priority, for example recent mild pain.

Although recent problem is technically the only general discriminator (Figure 2.8), the timeframes applied to each of these levels of acuteness are used throughout the charts:

- Abrupt is an onset within seconds or minutes
- Rapid onset is within 12 hours
- Acute indicates within 24 hours
- Recent is within the last 7 days

Any presentation beyond the 'recent' within 7 days and in the absence of any other discriminators would result in a priority 5 (blue) outcome. The use of this discriminator is not intended to 'punish' patients for an 'inappropriate' attendance, nor is it intended to ensure that patients who have had injuries or illnesses for a long time have extended waiting times. The actual waiting time for patients, with stable problems not of recent onset, will depend on the current case mix and case load of the department, and the resources available.

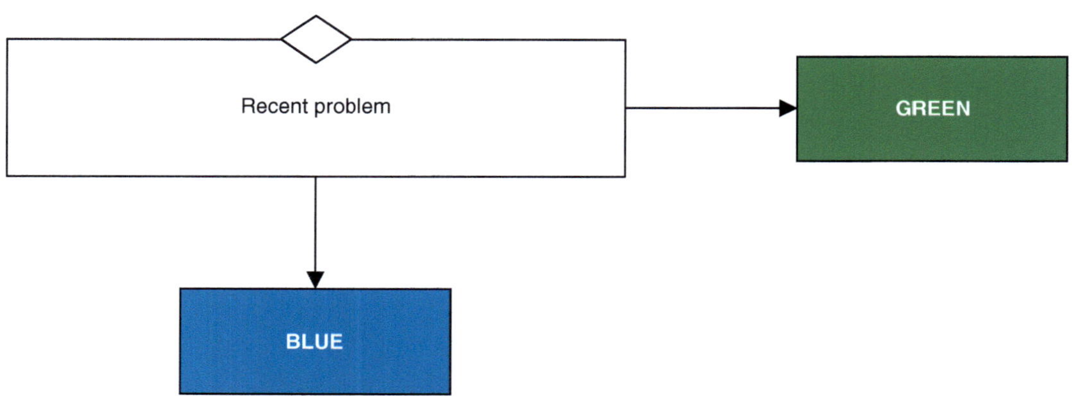

Figure 2.8 Acuteness

It is important to note that the chart in Figure 2.9 does not form one of the clinical patient presentation charts but is used for teaching purposes only.

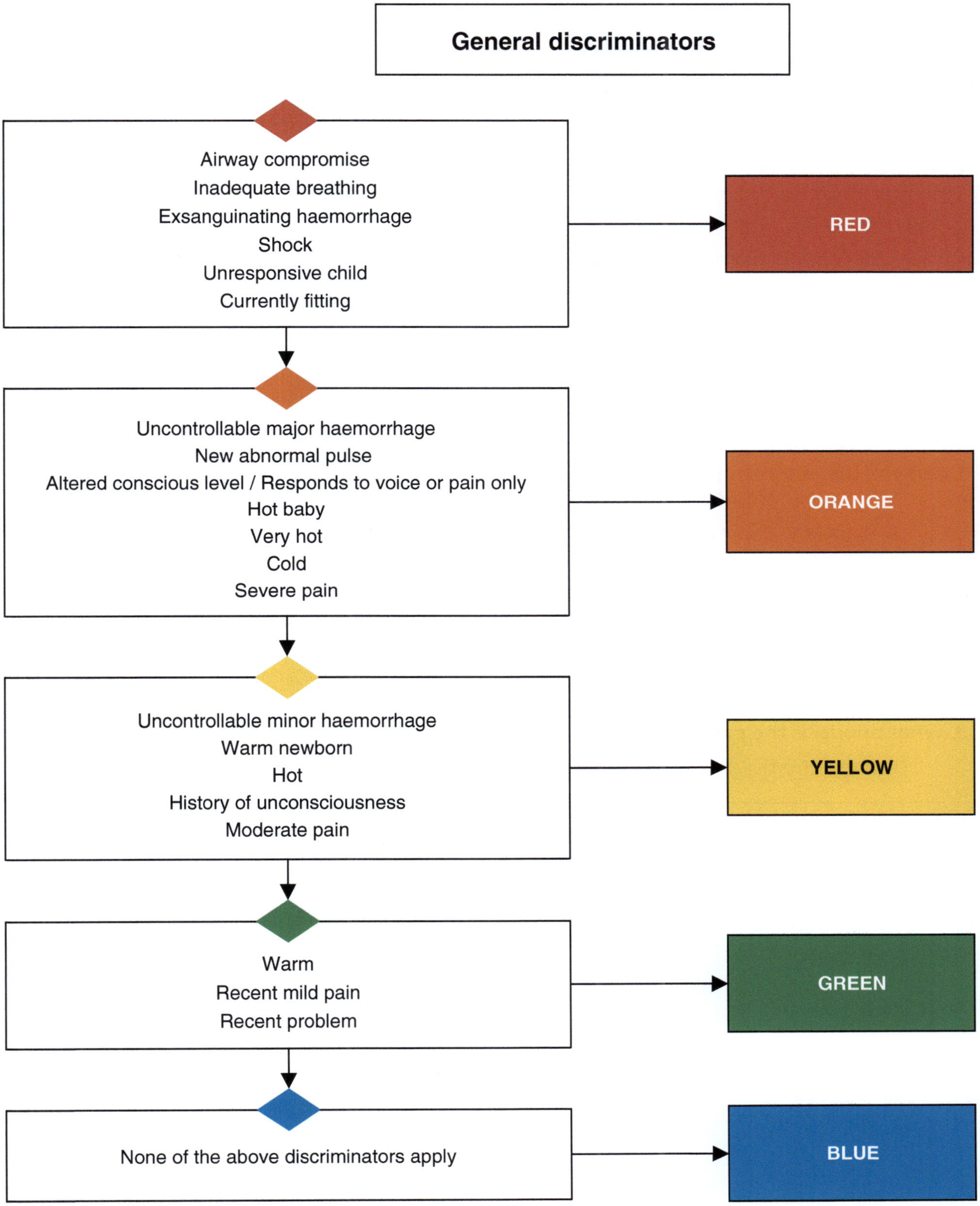

Figure 2.9 General discriminators

Evaluating all the alternatives and selecting the one for implementation

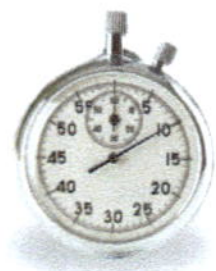

Time out exercise

Using only the general discriminator chart on page 17, try reviewing the following case studies and select the highest order discriminator to reach a priority for each one.

Case study 2.1

- A 95-year-old woman found lying unresponsive on the bedroom floor by her daughter
- Cyanosed
- RR 30 (shallow) breaths per minute
- Pulse 126 beats per minute
- Oxygen saturation = 72% on air
- GCS 6

Questions:

1. Can you triage the patient from the information provided?
   - What questions do you need to ask?

     Is the patient's airway patent, is the patient breathing?
     Cyanosed
     RR 30 (shallow) breaths per minute

2. Using the general discriminator chart, what is the highest order discriminator that applies to this patient?

   Airway compromise

3. What priority is the patient?

   Priority 1 (red)

Case study 2.2

- A 22-year-old man presents with a 3-day history of toothache
- He is not registered with a dentist
- Increasing pain today and facial swelling
- Temperature 36.6°C
- He states his pain is moderate

Questions:

1. Can you triage the patient from the information provided?
    - What questions do you need to ask?

    None of the red discriminators apply to this patient
    In orange we need to assess pain as none of the other higher order discriminators apply
    Temperature 36.6°C
    Increasing pain today and facial swelling
    Patient reports moderate pain

2. Using the general discriminator chart, what is the highest order discriminator that applies to this patient?

    Moderate pain

3. What priority is the patient?

    Priority 3 (yellow)

Implementing the selected alternative

Specific discriminators

Specific discriminators are applicable to individual presentations or to small groups of presentations and tend to relate to key features of certain conditions. Thus, while severe pain is a general discriminator, cardiac pain and pleuritic pain are specific discriminators. Choosing the most applicable chart is essential for accurate triage using the MTS. Selecting a chart mainly populated by general discriminators such as collapse, falls, unwell adult, unwell child or unwell baby, when there is evidently a more specific chart that matches the patient presentation, is likely to result in missing important relevant discriminators and may potentially lead to the wrong priority being allocated.

Specific discriminators also convey an important message to the next clinician who views the triage record, which is why selecting the highest order discriminator, most specific to the patient presentation, is an essential component of the MTS. As an example, consider the discriminators moderate pain and frank haematuria – both appear in priority 3 (yellow) but the latter denotes important information to any receiving clinician as many patients may be priority 3 (yellow) where moderate pain was their only applicable discriminator.

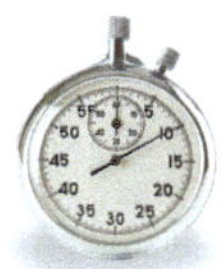

Time out exercise

Using one specific patient presentation flowchart, from the 54 listed, attempt to triage the following case study, selecting the highest order discriminator and priority.

Case study 2.3

- A 14-year-old girl attends having fallen onto her right knee whilst running for a bus
- She felt a sudden sharp pain in her knee
- Reduced range of movement in her right leg and evident bruising
- Unable to extend her right leg or straight leg raise and only able to partially weight bear
- She states that she has Von Willebrand disease
- She assesses her pain score as moderate

Questions:

1. Can you triage the patient from the information provided?

   Choose the most specific chart, which is limb problems

2. Using all the discriminators in the chosen chart, what is the highest order discriminator that applies to this patient?

   Bleeding disorder (defined as 'Congenital or acquired bleeding disorder')

3. What priority is the patient?

   Priority 3 (yellow)

In this case study we have established an important specific discriminator for this patient relating to bleeding disorder due to her Von Willebrand disease. If only general discriminators had been used she would still have been priority 3 (yellow) but the discriminator moderate pain would apply and as a result crucial information about the patient and her injury would have been omitted.

The discriminator dictionary

Each of the 203 discriminators comes with its own definition that can be found in the discriminator dictionary alphabetically listed at the end of the book. When using the MTS it is important to always have access to the discriminator dictionary as a quick reference guide. When triage practitioners are learning the system, they need to frequently refer to the definitions, ensuring they are making decisions based on the same detail all other triage practitioners are using. For more experienced clinicians there may be discriminators that are infrequently used and again sense checking the definition is an important patient safety feature of MTS.

The facing pages of each presentation flowchart details the specific discriminators listed for ease of reference, but there will be other discriminators in the charts that are contained within the main dictionary only. All discriminators are reviewed for each edition and version with updates of all changes published on the triage website: **www.triagenet.net**.

Monitoring the implementation and evaluating outcome

Clinical priority can change and triage must therefore be dynamic. The triage method described can be carried out rapidly and reliably by qualified clinicians; it is therefore useful as a tool for multiple re-evaluations of clinical priority during the patient's stay.

Every encounter can be used as a triage assessment and any change in clinical priority can be rapidly notified and acted upon.

CHAPTER 3

The triage event

Introduction

The Manchester Triage System (MTS) is designed to guide the triage practitioner's decision making to rapidly assign a clinical priority for each patient. To make the most effective use of the patient interaction, practitioners need to be confident and competent to perform a triage consultation. The assessment must always be structured, systematic and reproducible, with the various aspects of the triage event pieced together to give a complete picture of the patient's presenting problem.

Before detailing the process of the triage event, it is important to set the scene and look at those factors that can significantly impact how triage practitioners' function and perform, namely the environment in which they practise triage and their preparedness to take on the role.

The triage environment

The ideal triage environment would consist of a dedicated area located at patient entrances, that is spacious, uncluttered, and equipped with everything needed to support rapid triage. In practice, however, the triage area is often a repurposed space that is far from ideal for conducting this important function. When considering how best to design a triage area the following factors are useful:

- Spacious enough to provide easy access for patients, especially those on ambulance trolleys, in wheelchairs, using walking aids or children in prams
- An uncluttered, tidy and well-organised environment
- All necessary equipment to hand and regularly restocked, for example dressings, slings, equipment for recording vital signs and analgesia

Adopting a linear process is highly beneficial, moving only from left to right to perform the triage assessment rather than behind and in front of a desk. Stand facing the MTS charts (visualised in paper format or on a computer), with the patient directly to one side, which means only one step is required to be next to the patient. This reduces the amount of movement required and speeds up the triage event (Figure 3.1).

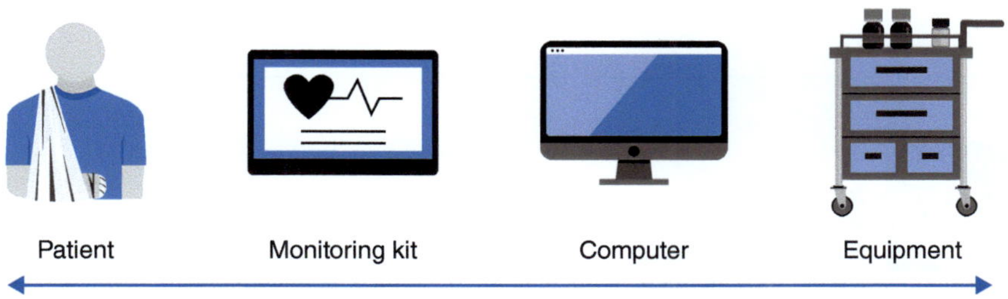

Figure 3.1 Linear triage process

Experience

Triage is a skilled role, undertaken for the most part unsupervised and often isolated from colleagues. For this reason, the triage practitioner requires sufficient experience of urgent and emergency care, alongside the interpersonal skills to communicate effectively with patients, families and carers. Whilst the MTS does not stipulate an exact amount of time before staff can be trained at provider level, experience is the key priority to commencing the training and supervision to confidently and competently undertake this important role. On average, services report around 18 months to 2 years' experience is required, but there are many variations, with others training more junior staff within 6–12 months after starting their careers.

To help shape the decision as to when triage training is appropriate, the following criteria are recommended. Before being considered for MTS provider level training candidates should:

1. Know their red flags – ensuring they can recognise and act appropriately to any life-threatening emergencies that can present at triage
2. Have gained foundation level experience in their specialty and to have achieved competence in all aspects of the service. In the UK, completing the Royal College of Nursing (RCN) Level 1 Career and Competency Framework is strongly recommended. Other specialties such as acute medicine also provide competencies to draw on. Newly qualified practitioners rarely achieve this level of competence in less than 12 months; in the first 6 months they should focus on preceptorship, allowing time to begin applying recently acquired knowledge and skills
3. Have composite knowledge and understanding of the patient journey. It is vital that triage practitioners know the back door management of a patient journey before being responsible for the front door (triage)
4. Be able to perform under the stringent supervision of a current MTS instructor after completing the provider course. This process is where they will be assessed and signed off as confident and competent to triage independently

The framework of triage assessment

The purist view of the triage event is a rapid and focused encounter in which information is gathered and applied to assign a priority. It is important that the assessment of a patient is systematic, with all elements of that assessment pieced together to provide a coherent picture of the patient's problem. The following framework should be used to ensure decisions are based on relevant and appropriate patient data.

Essentially there are four main components to the triage event that practitioners need to pay attention to:

- What you see
- What you hear
- What you do
- What you feel

What you see

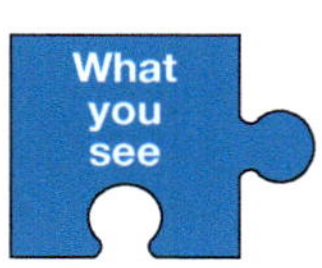

Observing the patient is an essential first step in the triage assessment and begins as soon as they come into view. So much valuable information can be gleaned before the patient even enters the triage area. Triage practitioners need to look at the patient as they approach, observing their behaviour, picking up on visual signs that may include the patient's level of mobility and movement, any obvious signs of illness, injury or pain and age of the patient.

Triage practitioners should actively observe patients within the waiting area, which constitutes their area of clinical responsibility. That responsibility applies to patients waiting to be triaged and those returned to this area post triage. The triage practitioner should never sit in their room and shout the patient's name; they need to regularly view the waiting area, constantly picking up information.

What you hear

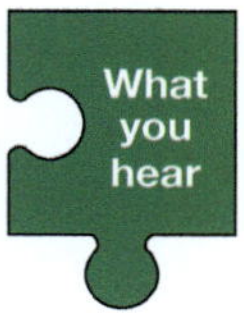

Asking focused questions and listening to responses during the triage event is where the practitioner's knowledge and skills are most evident and where experience makes a real difference. Once the patient provides the initial subjective history, the most specific presentation flowchart can be selected.

The focused questions are guided by each of the discriminators within the chart. Systematically working down the priorities (reductionist methodology), triage practitioners use this framework of questions until the first higher order discriminator that applies to the patient is reached. However, the chart is not a mere check list, the MTS is a clinical tool and the use of clinical knowledge to interpret the discriminators and the information being provided is essential in this professional system.

As well as using discriminators to focus questions, further clarification is often required. This may take the form of obtaining more details, for example mechanism of injury, duration of the problem or current medications.

> The MTS framework is designed to guide the practitioner's decision making, ensuring the triage event is systematic and not a series of random questions and actions. There should be no unstructured lengthy conversations with the patient or exhaustive history taking prior to the selection of the most specific presentation flowchart. Once selected, the chart dictates the format of the focused questions until the priority is identified.

Time out exercise

To review the first part of the triage process, 'what you see and what you hear', carefully look at the photograph of a triage handover and consider what is wrong with this picture (Figure 3.2). Make a short list of the issues identified and then review the points in Table 3.1.

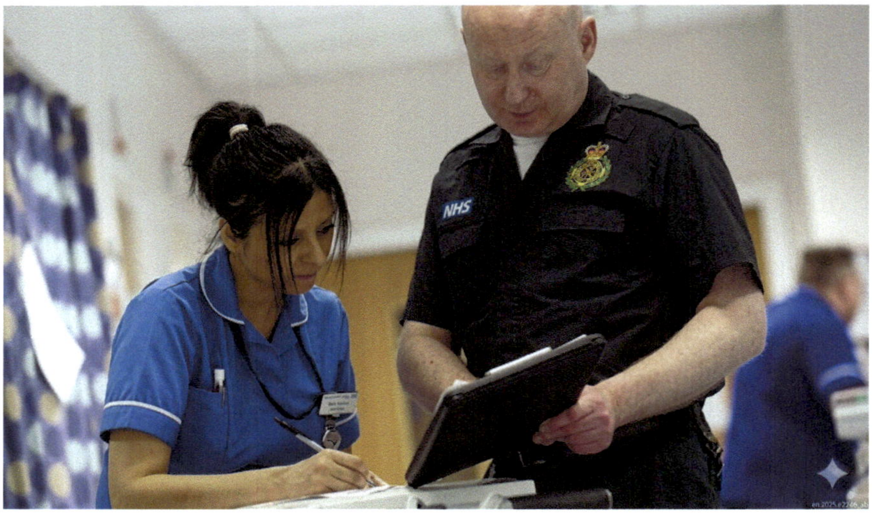

Figure 3.2 Source: Royal College of Nursing / https://rcni.com/emergency-nurse/evidence-and-practice/cpd-articles / last accessed May 1, 2026

Table 3.1 Issues identified

Identified issue from the photograph	**MTS discussion on ensuring a safe reliable and reproducible triage event**
Where is the patient?	MTS is a face-to-face triage system – there is no visualisation of any patient in the photograph **Remember: face to face every time** –always triage the patient unless the patient lacks capacity. Do not rely on second hand information, including that from pre-hospital personnel, when the patient is able to respond to your focused questions (as indicated by the discriminators in the selected chart)
The patient is not involved in the triage event	If the patient has capacity, why are you not triaging them? Ambulatory or ambulance conveyance is subject to the same principle – always attempt triage with the patient first and foremost
No visualisation of the MTS chart	There must always be easy access to, and use of, the full suite of MTS presentation flowcharts and discriminators. Choosing the most specific chart and using the decision-making framework to guide the questions and actions required ensures safe, reliable and reproducible triage decisions **Remember: chart to view every time.** Work down the discriminators until the highest order discriminator that applies to the patient is reached
Poor documentation using paper/notepad	Patient data should not be written on notepads, etc. Direct input onto a triage form (manual) or computerised system ensures accuracy of data capture and reduces the time to document the triage event

What you do

Vital signs and the appropriateness

Within each of the presentation flowcharts certain actions are indicated, the most commonplace being the recording of vital signs. The MTS works on the principle that observations are found in the charts when observations are required. This is opposed to a blanket approach where a full set of observations must be recorded on all patients, as this action regularly includes many perfectly healthy patients who do not require having their vital signs recorded.

The illness-related charts contain a range of observations, in the form of discriminators, for example very low oxygen saturation, temperature ranges or new abnormal pulse. The time taken to complete vital sign recording in these cases is important as it presents the triage practitioner with another piece of the information required to safely prioritise the patient. In contrast, when a patient presents with a simple limb injury, minor laceration or a foreign body lodged in their ear, vital signs are not indicated and for good reasons. However, sometimes a degree of common sense is required – the charts indicate where vital signs should be recorded, but the triage practitioner may decide certain patients would also benefit from this action. As an example, in a patient presenting with sudden/acute loss or altered vision, recording a blood pressure to check for hypertension would be indicated.

Monitoring of physiological parameters

Triage is a dynamic process and should be undertaken periodically on all patients while they are waiting for treatment. In this way any change in status can be identified and the triage category modified if necessary. The need for monitoring does not stop after first clinician contact. It is important that any deterioration is identified as soon as possible so that appropriate reassessment can be undertaken and any treatments started. The similarity between post triage monitoring (dynamic triage) and post clinical assessment monitoring is self-evident.

Many services have adopted an 'early warning score' format and in some areas of the hospital this has been successful. However, in urgent and emergency care the discriminators within the MTS, particularly those addressing the ABCD life threat, lend themselves well to ongoing assessment and can easily be adapted into an early warning tool (Table 3.2). The use of these MTS-based physiological parameters ensures clinicians are familiar with the process and can quickly identify deterioration (or improvement) in the patient's condition.

Table 3.2 MTS ABCD discriminators

	Red	Orange	Yellow
Airway	Airway compromise		
Breathing	Inadequate breathing	Very low SpO_2 Unable to talk in sentences	Low SpO_2
Circulation	Shock Exsanguinating haemorrhage	New abnormal pulse Tachycardia in children Uncontrollable major haemorrhage	Uncontrollable minor haemorrhage
Disability	Unresponsive child Hypoglycaemia	Altered conscious level	History of unconsciousness

As with all monitoring tools, it is change rather than absolute score that is important. Thus, the new appearance of a red discriminator should indicate immediate clinical reassessment, while the recognition of an orange or yellow discriminator should precipitate clinical action within 10 or 60 minutes, respectively. This approach has the advantage of using a tool with which triage practitioners are familiar, and within a framework that is well known.

Physical assessment at triage

On those occasions when an area of the body needs examination to move past a discriminator, for example assessment of a limb for gross deformity or checking the skin for any rash, this again needs to be performed as quickly and simply as possible. One such use would be when assessing upper and lower limb injuries to refer patients directly for radiological investigations. There is likely to be a reduction in the total time spent in the department if patients present to the treating clinician with radiographs ready for interpretation.

Analgesia at triage

There is real patient benefit to the assessment of pain and early administration of appropriate analgesia. Ensuring this procedure is easily facilitated within the triage environment is important. Any drugs administered at triage need to be safely stored in the triage room for rapid access, and the recording mechanisms, whether that be paper based or computerised, must also be quick and easy to complete.

First aid

Quick and simple first aid measures are important at triage, for example the application of a sling, pressure dressing or simple wound dressing.

What you feel

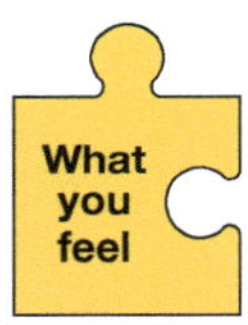

There will be certain patients assigned a priority as indicated by the MTS where the triage practitioner feels they need to be seen sooner by a clinician for a specific reason. There could be a patient safety issue or they may require interim treatment, for example a nebuliser. In these cases, the triage priority should not be altered but post triage it is appropriate to expedite patient management using streaming, fast track protocols or simply relaying concerns to another clinician.

Putting the pieces together

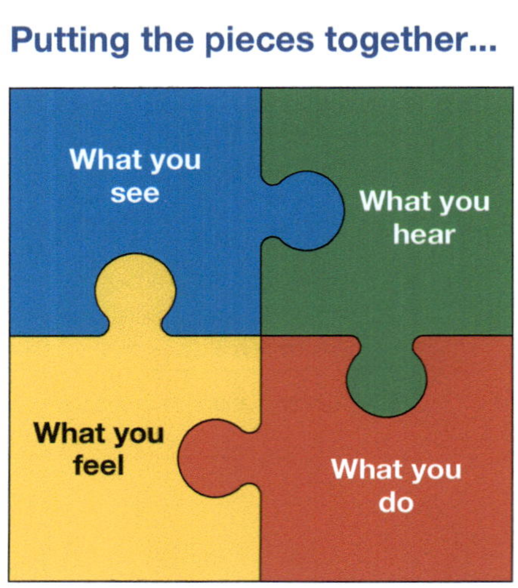

The following exercise shows how the triage event would progress to a conclusion using the systematic process of the MTS framework.

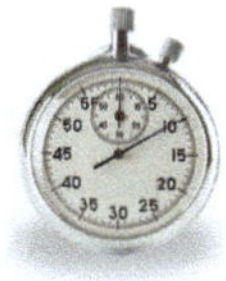

Time out exercise

Case study 3.1

A 54-year-old-man attends having wrenched his right shoulder pushing a truck with work colleagues.

Questions:

- Which presentational flowchart will you choose?

  Limb problems – review this chart (page 128), the discriminators and definitions to enhance understanding of the process before continuing with this exercise

- What questions do you need to ask?

  Make sure to follow the reductionist methodology
  Any ABCD life threat? The patient is walking and talking – therefore not a red priority

- Review the orange discriminators

  He felt a sudden sharp pain in his shoulder and upper arm
  Reduced range of movement in shoulder
  Unable to abduct right arm due to pain

- Pain assessment. The final orange discriminator requires assessment of his pain

  He assesses his pain score as mild – therefore not an orange priority

- Review the yellow discriminators

  None of the yellow discriminators apply – therefore not a yellow priority

- Review the green discriminators

  Some swelling to the shoulder
  Mild pain

- Can you assign a priority?
- Which highest order discriminator applies?

Case outcome

Chart	Limb problems
Discriminator	Swelling
Priority	Green (priority 4)

Documenting the triage event

Both manual and computerised versions of the MTS are successfully used across the world. There are specifications for computerised systems that can be found on **Triagenet.net** but essentially any triage documentation should be designed to promote rapid completion. The triage method allows documentation to be simple and precise. The minimum data required are a record of the chosen presentation flowchart, the discriminator selected and the priority associated with that particular discriminator. Thus, for instance, the triage record of a patient with chest pain might be:

- Chest pain
- Pleuritic pain
- Yellow (priority 3)
- *Free text section*

Ideally the triage document should mirror the MTS framework, with quick access to data fields where vital signs can be recorded as they are taken, without having to move to other documents or opening more computer tabs. This simple approach to documentation also facilitates simple audit.

Triage assessment procedure

Assessment component	Triage activity
Greeting the patient What you see 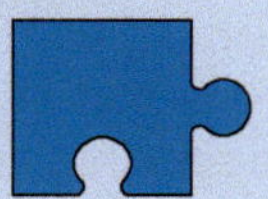	The assessment begins at first sight of the patient; watch the patient as they approach the triage area and pick up on any visual signs, which may include: • Level of mobility • Obvious illness/injury • Age of patient
Patient's history What you hear 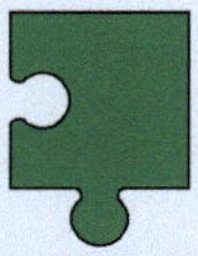	Ask the patient why they have attended the service This is a short, concise, subjective history and tells you about the patient's injury/illness/health-related problem
Presenting complaint	The patient's presenting complaint is established from the short subjective history they provide, leading the triage practitioner to choose the most specific presentation flowchart
Focused questions What you hear 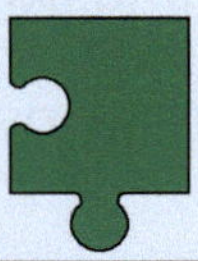	**Focused questions are directed by the discriminators** in the chosen presentation flowchart. More detail may be required in the form of clarification questions, e.g. mechanism of injury, duration of the problem, current medications, etc.
Physical examination and assessment of physical parameters What you do 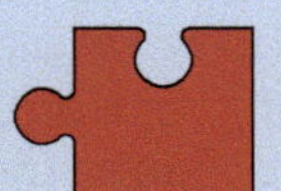	Vital signs only appear in the charts where observations are required. Rapid physical assessment is indicated where necessary to identify signs and symptoms First aid administered
Pain assessment and administration of analgesia	This is an integral part of the MTS, where both patient (subjective) and triage practitioner (objective) pain scores are recorded. Any variance between the two scores will be justified using the behavioral objectives
Documentation	The recording of this information should be in an agreed format which is clear, concise and provides specific information to inform the next clinician accessing the patient's triage record When a computerised triage system is in place, the triage practitioner should make sure the focus of attention is always the patient and not the computer screen/keyboard
Priority/plan of care What you feel 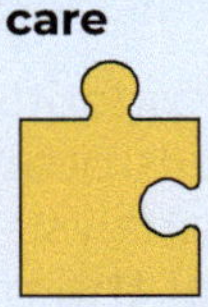	A clinical priority is assigned using the highest order discriminator applicable to the patient Give a brief description of any further care identified as a result of the triage assessment Patient streamed to appropriate area of the service – making good use of a streaming tool such as the presentation priority matrix (PPM)
Reassessment	Document where there is a need to reassess and the reason why. Record the new priority

Free text

The addition of a free text section is another important feature of the triage document and offers practitioners the opportunity to add clear, concise and specific information to inform the next clinician who accesses the triage record. The key to purposeful free text is firstly making sure there is not too much erroneous detail, avoiding content that is not specific to this presentation. There can be a temptation to write out all the negative findings that were discriminated for as the practitioner moved down the chart. It is likely the only purposeful negative finding worthy of note is 'no loss of consciousness' (no LOC). It is important to ensure that appropriate details are included, and vital information is not omitted, such as relevant previous medical history and medications.

Achieving and sustaining rapid triage

From the outset, the MTS was designed as a rapid, focused assessment and allocation of priority, taking on average just 2–3 minutes. The MTS is undoubtedly one of the best risk assessment tools at the point of entry to urgent and emergency care. However, this risk can only be quantified and mitigated if all patients are triaged quickly and effectively. An appropriate standard for the maximum time most patients should wait for triage would be within 15 minutes of their arrival. The reality is that if triage events take longer than 5 minutes a queue of patients quickly forms. The result of any time delay is an unknown risk for all those patients waiting for triage, some of whom will be presenting with significant health problems.

The complete triage event needs to be a 'pit stop' – fast and focused – rather than an 'MOT' (motor ordinance test) which is slow and detailed. Using the Formula One analogy of a pit stop that takes seconds is useful in instilling the idea that the triage event is time pressured, and rapidly completed through a structured and repetitive process. In contrast, an MOT is detailed, slow and takes many hours.

Interestingly, audit has demonstrated that the average triage intervention time is between 60 and 120 seconds, which contradicts any notion that the MTS slows down the triage process. An excellent example of the most efficient use of MTS is seen in emergency departments across Portugal where the average triage time is a mere 90 seconds per patient. There are now over 25 years of data from Portugal that demonstrate this excellent standard; not only have they made this amazing achievement, but it has remained consistent. It is also worthy of note that Portuguese triage nurses reliably demonstrate the most precise and consistent levels of accuracy (>97%) using the MTS, as seen from data reported monthly as part of the national audit process in every public, private and military hospital.

The reality is that triage events are slowed down due to tasks other than prioritisation which are carried out by triage practitioners as part of the assessment. For example, electrocardiography (ECG), which can take more than 10 minutes to complete, cannulation and blood analysis and lengthy risk assessments, none of which are required to assign a clinical priority. One of the major frustrations expressed by triage practitioners is the sheer volume of duties not related to triage that they are expected to complete during this patient event. These extra tasks often provide minimal patient benefit, yet they are placed in triage simply because doing so guarantees they will be completed.

These added tasks would be acceptable at this stage of the patient's journey if there were enough triage practitioners working at any one time to ensure that no patient waited more than 15 minutes before being triaged, but rarely is this the case. It may not be possible, or indeed appropriate, to carry out all the assessments necessary at the initial triage encounter, particularly when the workload of the service is high. In such circumstances the necessary assessments should still be carried out, but as secondary procedures by another member of the team, for example recording an ECG for a patient presenting with cardiac pain.

To improve efficiency and quality of the triage event it is highly recommended that a lean methodology is adopted. Applying these principles, it is possible to identify and strip out unnecessary non-triage-based activities with the aim of dramatically improving triage times and, as a result, patient safety (see Further reading).

Stressing the higher priorities

Patient management is not the same as MTS priority and under no circumstances should a patient priority be manipulated to meet local or national targets, to favour specific age groups or clinical conditions or to meet key performance indicators. Examples of where services inappropriately alter an MTS priority, and confuse this with departmental management, include:

1. The diktat that all patients with a fractured neck of femur must be given an orange priority.
2. The rule that all patients over 70 with a given frailty score must be seen within 10 minutes (orange priority).
3. The rule that after 2200 hours all children under the age of 5 years must be seen within 10 minutes (orange priority).

There are many examples where this manipulation results in seriously stressing a particular priority, often the very urgent/orange priority. The result of this inappropriate activity is that patients who are rightly triaged orange (according to MTS methodology) experience extended delays for their management, resulting in increased risk of patient harm.

To reduce the temptation of merely assigning whole patient groups to a particular priority, the answer comes in the form of post triage streaming, not manipulating the triage process (see Chapter 5). Using the patient group presenting with a fractured neck of femur as an example, there will be a range of priorities allocated, some may be orange due to severe pain, but many will be yellow due to gross deformity or moderate pain. The priority, as indicated by the MTS, should be accurately documented. Any further action required to meet a key performance indicator, such as all these patients must be admitted within a specific timeframe, is achieved through the streaming process. Streaming will invoke the use of specific pathways of care to expedite the management of this group of patients.

The result of inappropriate priority allocation is a significant skewing of the patient case mix where it appears more patients are in higher priorities than is actually the case. Manipulation of priority is not only an issue for those patients who are rightly in that category, but it also makes any attempt to audit triage unreliable.

Never confuse departmental management with patient priority. There should not be any blanket application whereby all patients with a particular problem, age, etc. are placed in a predetermined triage priority. Rather, their journey can be expedited during the streaming process post triage.

Managing the waiting room

Until a patient has been seen by a clinician, the patient's main contact is the triage practitioner. Constant observation and reassessment are necessary to identify those patients whose condition is changing. Triage is a dynamic process, and patients often need regular reassessment. No one can anticipate all problems, and it is not a 'failure' of accurate assessment to change the triage category according to further developments in the patient's condition, or indeed with further information that may be acquired. The waiting room should be considered a clinical area and the domain and responsibility of the triage practitioner.

Re-triage

Triage is a dynamic process and should not be seen as an isolated incident that only occurs at the beginning of the patient's journey. The triage practitioner must use their decision-making skills and expertise to identify those patients requiring ongoing monitoring and potential re-triage. For example, a patient could be reprioritised after administration of adequate analgesia and subsequent pain relief, or after a negative ECG finding reprioritised from orange to yellow or even a green priority. It should be noted that re-triage can result in both increasing and decreasing a priority as appropriate to that patient presentation.

It is likely that re-triage activity occurs more often than thought but the process is not always accurately recorded. When re-triage is indicated and subsequent reprioritising occurs, the change must be recorded in the patient documentation and accompanied by the reason for the new priority.

Summary

The MTS framework provides a structured, systematic and reproducible approach to the triage assessment and should take the format shown on page 31.

By following the systematic process, facilitated by the MTS framework, triage can be performed rapidly and confidently to reach an appropriate clinical priority in order to guide decision making.

CHAPTER 4

Pain assessment as part of the triage process

Pain assessment at triage

Pain is a key issue for patients attending urgent and emergency care and is often their main focus. Pain assessment has improved significantly since the first edition of *Emergency Triage*; however, it needs to remain at the forefront of the triage event so that pain continues to be assessed and managed appropriately.

There are several factors affecting why pain is an important issue:

- The majority of patients attending urgent and emergency care present with some degree of pain
- The degree of pain influences the urgency
- Unmediated pain can increase in severity
- Patients in pain can become agitated and aggressive
- Patients in pain are a source of distress and stress to both staff and other patients
- The adequacy of pain management is a key criterion for patient satisfaction
- Patients have an expectation that their pain will be dealt with

There are many advantages in assessing pain as part of the triage process. Firstly, it ensures that a patient's pain is managed at the earliest opportunity and that appropriate analgesia is provided. A consequent reduction in pain may lead to the possibility of re-triage to a lower priority. Secondly, patient anxiety is reduced, often leading to improved communication. Without pain assessment the provision of appropriate analgesia at triage is not possible.

If a patient's pain is to be assessed formally at triage, and the outcome of that assessment used to determine the urgency with which that patient is to be seen, then all triage practitioners must be competent in assessing pain, and the pain assessment must be valid and reproducible. Training triage practitioners in pain assessment, the use of a valid pain assessment tool and important considerations when assessing pain are all aspects of the Manchester Triage System (MTS) Provider Course, designed to improve knowledge, develop confidence and competence.

The ideal pain assessment tool

An ideal pain tool should be quick and simple to use, should have been validated and must provide reliable, reproducible results. It is common practice for urgent and emergency care services to use a formal pain assessment tool, but many such tools suffer from the fact that they were developed for use with postoperative and chronically ill patients.

There are three main types of pain assessment tools:

- Verbal descriptor scales
- Visual analogue scales
- Pain behaviour tools

Verbal descriptor scales

These scales consist of word descriptors, usually three to five, which are ranked with the value increasing in line with the severity of the pain. The most common descriptors include:

- None
- Slight
- Moderate
- Severe
- Excruciating

The verbal descriptor scale is short and relatively easy for most patients to use and has been employed in the emergency care environment (Table 4.1).

Table 4.1 The verbal descriptor scale

Advantages	Disadvantages
Provides a score that is easy for any practitioner to analyse	The use of a single word from a limited list may not accurately reflect the pain that the patient is experiencing
Probably produces reliable data	It is not suitable for patients who do not speak the common language
Can be modified for use in children	It is the patient's subjective assessment

Visual analogue scales

These scales usually consist of a straight line representing varying levels of pain with verbal anchors at each end.

NO PAIN	**PAIN AS BAD AS IT COULD BE**

Patients can mark anywhere on the line and verbal descriptors can also be added beneath the line in addition to the word anchors. The line can also be broken down to facilitate scoring of pain. Numerical scores are often expressed from 0 to 10, with 0 representing no pain and 10 being excruciating (Table 4.2).

Table 4.2 The visual analogue scale

Advantages	Disadvantages
Easy and fast to use and score	Some patients choose to mark the line near one of the verbal anchors
These scales may be more sensitive than verbal descriptors	Certain patients find these scales too abstract to use, in particular those in severe pain, those with learning disabilities or those with impaired motor coordination
When used correctly they are reproducible and reliable	The elderly can also have some difficulty in using these scales

Pain behaviour tools

These tools have been developed relying on the principle that patients who are in pain exhibit certain behaviours and physiological changes. These tools can measure the following:

- Verbal response
- Body language
- Facial expression
- Behavioural changes
- Conscious level
- Physiological changes

Pain behaviours

Simple, descriptive terms can be used by clinicians to assess patient pain behaviours, for example:

- Normal activities – no pain/mild pain
- A few problems – can do most things – mild pain
- Causes difficulties – stops some things – moderate pain
- Disabling – stops normal activities – severe pain
- No control – severe pain

Many different tools exist, each based on combining several of the factors listed but have some disadvantages in use (Table 4.3).

Table 4.3 The pain behaviour tool

Advantages	Disadvantages
Can be used in patients with communication problems	Complex scales can make comparison and scoring difficult and time consuming, taking 5–15 minutes to use The patient's subjective assessment is not included Difficult to ensure that pain alone underlies the observed behavioural changes

The pain ruler

No single pain assessment tool is better than another, although some would seem to be more suited to specific clinical areas than others. The pain ruler is a well-established pain assessment tool that lends itself for use in urgent and emergency care settings. In particular, its advantages are that it:

- Measures the intensity of pain and the effects on normal function
- Combines the use of verbal descriptor and visual analogue scales
- Is fast and easy to use
- Is easily weighted to allow pain assessment to be part of the triage process
- Facilitates the use of pain behaviours to strengthen both patient and clinician pain scoring
- Promotes dialogue, which in turn encourages patients that their pain is being taken seriously
- Produces a score, facilitating ongoing assessment to track improvement or deterioration
- Ensures the outcome of the assessment is quick and easy to document
- Can easily be adapted for use in children

The pain ruler offers scores of 0–10 with sections grouped into no pain, mild pain, moderate pain and severe pain, which is congruent with other pain scoring tools. The same group of descriptions are used as general discriminators in the presentation flowcharts. A pain ruler is shown in Figure 4.1.

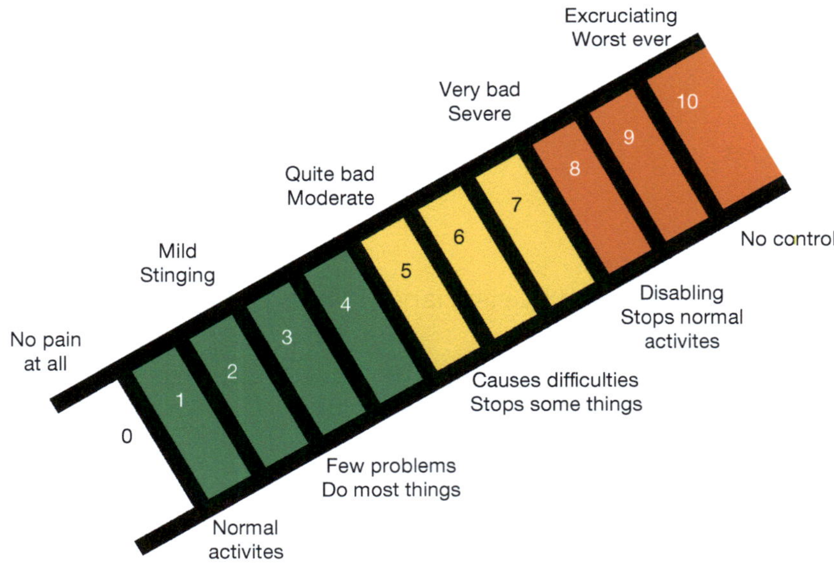

Figure 4.1 Pain ruler

The pain ruler can easily be supplemented with a faces scale for use in younger children as shown in Figure 4.2.

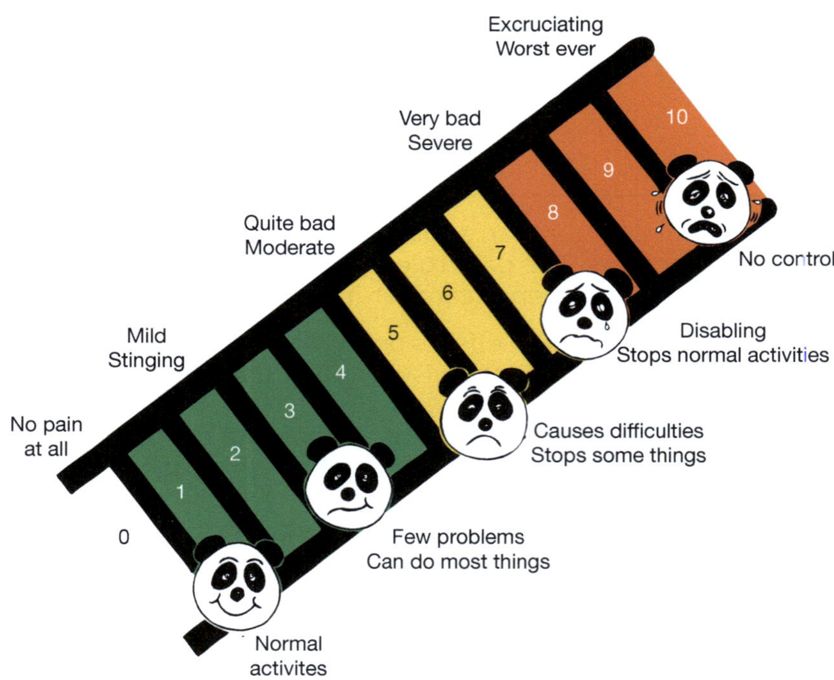

Figure 4.2 Faces scale pain ruler for use in younger children

An alternative, easy to use, pain assessment tool

One of the main problems with the pain ruler is the perceived complexity by some patients and clinicians. As a visual tool it can be quickly understood but the patient needs to be looking at the picture and in practice the pain ruler is often quickly described to the patient but rarely shown. To simplify the pain assessment for patients, switching to a more purposeful question, that requires little or no explanation, can be achieved by asking the patient:

'Do you think your pain is MILD, MODERATE or SEVERE?'

This quick and easy question means the patient effectively has three possible choices. The pain ruler can be easily adapted to match the simple question as it is split into sections representing mild, moderate and severe pain. As increasing numbers of services adopt this simple version, and anecdotal reports show a reduction in the variance between patient and triage practitioner pain scores, which could be a sign of more accurate pain assessment.

The importance of both patient (subjective) and clinician (objective) pain scores

Pain assessment is an integral part of the MTS methodology and represents a deliberate and explicit recognition of the importance of pain. It is recognised that the result of routinely assessing pain is that patients may be categorised as a higher priority than was traditionally the case. It is unrealistic to expect that only the patient's subjective assessment will be taken into consideration during a rapid triage pain assessment but it is equally inappropriate that triage practitioners make their own subjective assessment of the patient's pain in isolation.

The triage event is time pressured and designed to take only a few minutes and as a result patients have limited time to make a decision and accurately score their pain. A patient under pressure may say their pain is severe to justify their attendance, whilst some patients, particularly children and the elderly, may deny that they have pain to avoid having treatment or being admitted to hospital. Some practitioners' assessment and management of pain may be influenced by 'traditional' pathways of care. For example, patients with fractures are offered immediate analgesia, but patients with abdominal pain may not be offered analgesia until after a clinical assessment.

There may be concerns by staff that a patient will score pain higher if it is thought that this will result in quicker treatment, but the objective assessment of pain is built into the pain ruler in order to ameliorate this factor.

The pain assessment process

Once the triage practitioner has asked the patient about their pain, when they are given the opportunity to best describe and score their pain, this is classed as the patient (subjective) score. After recording the patient score, the triage practitioner then proceeds to enter data for the clinician (objective) pain score, which is reached by using the pain behaviours to assess and establish if these two scores match (Figure 4.3).

Within the MTS both these values are mandatory fields and if there is any difference between them there needs to be a justification recorded by the triage practitioner clearly stating the rationale for the variance.

Choosing which of the pain behaviours best matches the situation is the simplest and most effective means of recording variance. However, it is important to note that the additional use of data from the triage practitioner is not meant to downplay or reduce the patient's assessment but is more an effort to strengthen the decision making.

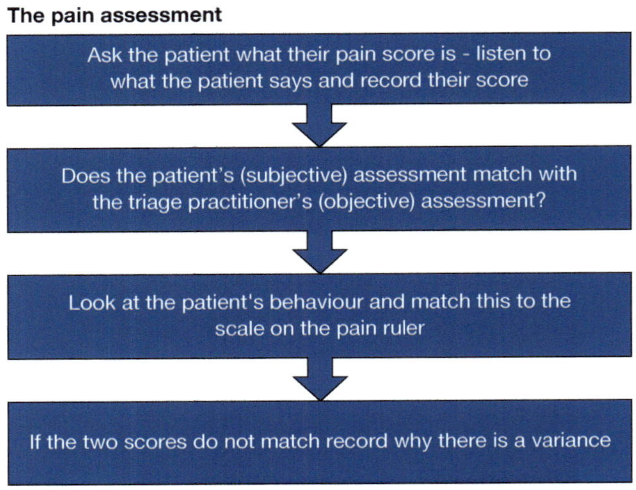

Figure 4.3 Pain assessment

Pain assessment is a skilled process in any environment and the assessment carried out during triage is no exception. There are constraints in this setting reflecting the emergency nature of the patient's condition and time critical characteristics of this assessment. Nevertheless, an accurate assessment of the patient's pain into one of the priorities shown in Figure 4.4 is essential if proper and timely care is to be given.

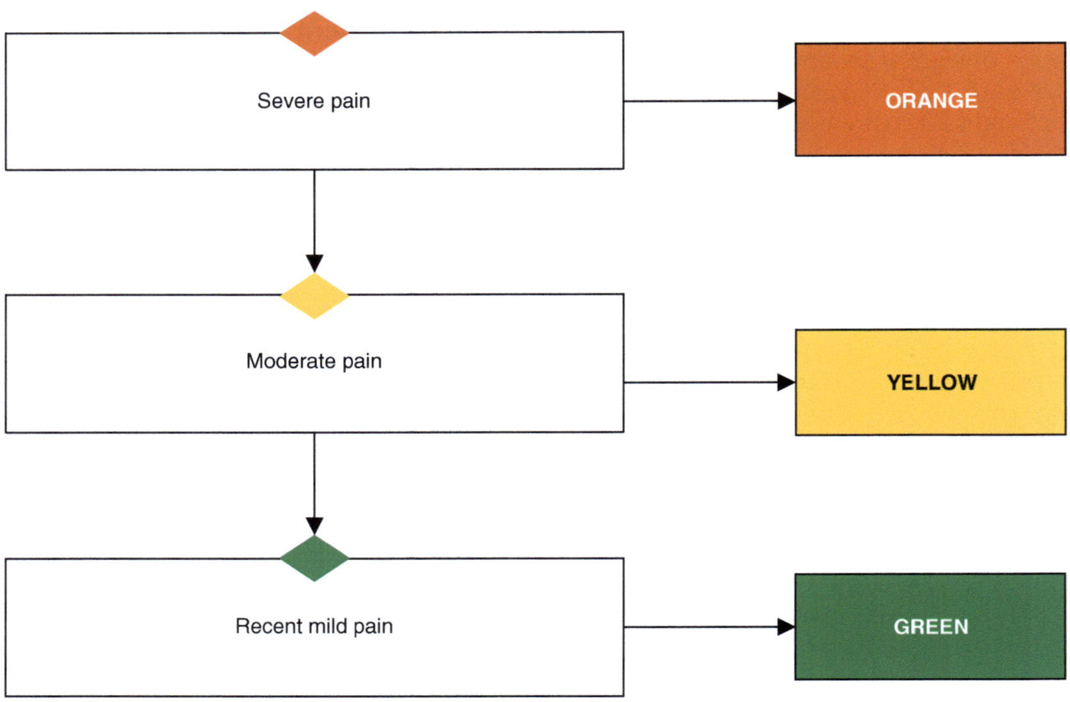

Figure 4.4 Pain priority categories

Factors influencing pain perception

During any pain assessment activity the triage practitioner must take into account a number of factors that influence a patient's perception of their pain.

Age

Children may imagine the worst possible outcome of their pain. They can employ catastrophic thinking which increases their anxiety and fear and may therefore enhance their perception of pain. The application of distraction techniques is a central skill of the triage practitioner and helps them distinguish pain from distress and anxiety. However, the assessment may take more time in children as developing rapport is essential for the accurate application of the pain tools. The triage practitioner must be able to recognise the signs of pain in pre- and non-verbal children and the pain ruler can be adapted by using a simple faces rating scale or the behavioural assessment: the face, legs, activity, cry and consolability (FLACC) scale.

At the opposite end of the life span, many elderly people suffer from persistent and complex pain issues. This patient group may underestimate severe pain as being moderate or even mild, making the use of the pain behaviour scale an important component of the triage practitioner's assessment in these cases. Many accept pain and appear to cope well with it, especially those that live their daily lives with a burden of pain, commonly musculoskeletal in nature, often assuming this as a normal part of ageing. Alternative pain assessment tools may be required for elderly patients who struggle to comprehend the pain ruler. Lack of comprehension may be due to a number of reasons: hearing or sight impairment, feeling too rushed to decide or impaired cognition. It is well understood that there is a direct correlation between impaired cognition and poor pain management and this presents another good case for using the more purposeful question that requires little or no explanation to accurately apply: 'Do you think your pain is mild, moderate or severe?'

There will be cases where patients have cognitive impairment and cannot engage in pain assessment, for example those with dementia, and in these cases specific tools should be employed, for example the pain assessment in advanced dementia (PAINAD) scale (based on FLACC) or the Abbey Pain Scale.

Assessment skill

- Recognise patients whose age affects pain assessment
- Consider whether pain perception is increased or decreased and how can this be overcome
- Understand what alternative pain tools may be required when lack of capacity prevents the accurate use of the pain ruler

Previous experience of pain

Patients are influenced by their previous experiences of pain but asking them to 'imagine the worst pain ever' is not a useful question. Everyone has a unique memory of their pain experiences and as a result their previous encounters are often an unreliable indicator. One person's experience of pain and the pain thresholds they can cope with will be entirely different to someone else's experience of pain. During the assessment it can sometimes be useful to have them compare this pain to previous episodes, if presenting with a recurring health problem, and whether the current pain is more or less severe.

Patients will also be influenced by how pain was previously managed and if they have a bad experience of poorly managed pain that memory can certainly heighten their anxiety. Alternatively, their previous experience may have resulted in the rapid administration of effective analgesia, and they will be expecting this to happen again during this event.

Assessment skill

- Recognise whether the patient has had similar pain before
- Consider what is different now
- Identify how the patient managed the pain previously

Culture

Illness behaviour, and therefore pain behaviour, has a strong cultural component, and because of different cultural and social influences not all individuals express pain in the same way. Pain behaviour continues to be reinforced throughout life by the social group to which the individual belongs.

Particular cultural groups do not feel pain less than others, but they can differ significantly in how they respond to, or express, their pain. It is essential triage practitioners recognise that their own cultural and social background will inevitably influence how they interpret a patient's pain behaviour. These cultural and social differences identify one particular difficulty with relying on assessment tools that consider only the patient's (or the practitioner's) subjective assessment.

Assessment skill

- Recognise your own and the patient's cultural background
- Consider how different cultures might affect the patient's pain perception
- Understand how different cultural responses to pain can affect the triage practitioner's interpretation of behaviour

Anxiety

There is a link between high anxiety levels and high pain scoring. Patients can be anxious for many reasons; they may be concerned about the effect of the illness/accident on their ability to carry out their everyday activities, and they may be anxious about attending hospital or worried about what is wrong with them. Dealing with anxiety is a unique response and everyone differs in how they cope with these emotions. Triage practitioners need to remain open minded when considering whether their patient's pain is heightened by anxiety.

It is now commonplace for people to turn to their mobile devices to help distract themselves when feeling stressed and anxious, therefore it is not acceptable to judge that a person 'playing on their phone' cannot be in pain. There are specific physical, mental health conditions and disabilities where patients are actively encouraged to use their mobile devices A perfect example of pain modulating behaviour can be found amongst the sickle cell and thalassaemia population, many of whom use apps designed to help reduce anxiety and attempt to modulate their pain. The same can be said for patients who have learning disabilities; apps can assist, and listening to music may help to calm patients and reduce pain, especially for individuals with autism. Physical movement may offer additional relief. In the case of children, they often react to the anxiety of their parents or carers and calming those attending with the patient means the child is more likely to be calm.

There are considerable benefits in addressing a patient's pain at triage, in that the patient is shown at the earliest opportunity their pain is being taken seriously. Pain can also be reduced just by relieving a patient of some of their anxieties, including dread and fear, by providing reassurance on what is likely to happen next. The key is good communication, reassurance and explanation from the triage practitioner which often plays an important part in effectively reducing the level of pain.

Assessment skill

- Recognise and acknowledge the patient's level of anxiety
- Consider what lies behind the patient's anxiety
- Try to establish if they have tried any methods to reduce their anxiety
- Consider how anxiety may affect the patient's perception of pain

Disruption to patient's usual activities

Each individual functions at a level they consider to be normal for them. Pain can destroy the patient's ability to perform at that level, affecting both physical and emotional well-being, their financial situation and their position within society. Patients' perception of their pain will be influenced to some extent by how the pain will stop them functioning normally. It may not be possible to fully assess the level of disruption to the patient's usual activities, but the triage practitioner may be able to help the patient to focus on the effect of the pain by asking pertinent questions, for example: 'Does the pain stop them from eating/drinking/sleeping/breathing properly?' 'Does the pain stop them walking/sitting?' and 'Does the pain stop them working/going to school?'

Assessment skill

- Recognise the degree to which normal daily activities are disrupted
- Understand how the degree of disruption can be assessed
- Consider how the degree of disruption relates to the patient's perception of pain

If a patient scores their pain as 10 but can perform all their usual activities, the practitioner should consider other factors that may be influencing the patient's assessment of their pain.

Other considerations

Some patients may not be able to participate in the pain assessment process. They may be confused, have severe learning disabilities or be too distressed to comply. Likewise, they may not be able to read or understand the spoken language. Consider each patient as an individual and think about other tools that need to be employed instead.

Assessment skill

- Recognise that no single assessment tool is appropriate for every patient presenting with pain
- Consider whether the patient can participate using this method of assessment
- Understand what other methods of pain assessment may be more appropriate

Time out exercise

Having reviewed this chapter, look at the following two case presentations (Table 4.4). Consider the difference in pain presentation and assessment against each of the pain behaviours listed.

Table 4.4 Comparison of two patient cases

Pain presentation and behaviours	Patient case 1	Patient case 2
Presenting complaint	A 62-year-old man presents with abdominal pain	A 23-year-old man presents with abdominal pain
History	He has a history of bowel cancer and has been treated with chemotherapy and radiotherapy over the past 10 months. He takes regular doses of opioids for pain control	He went out drinking with friends last night and woke this morning with lower abdominal pain and reports he has vomited twice
Body language	Doubled over in pain and has great difficulty walking to triage from the waiting room	Able to walk unaided, sitting comfortably in the chair
Facial expression	Looks pale, facial grimacing especially on any movement	Looks relaxed, smiling during triage event
Verbal responses	Has difficulty listening to and answering questions at triage, apologises but can only speak in short bursts of 2–3 words at a time as another wave of pain distracts him and he shouts out in pain	Talks in full sentences, able to listen to and answer all questions. Occasionally touches his lower abdomen
Patient (subjective) pain assessment	Indicates pain as moderate now as he has taken an extra dose of opioids before he left home	Indicates pain as severe, worst pain he has ever experienced
Physiological changes	Increased heart rate Increased respiratory rate Sweating profusely	All vital signs within normal limits
Triage practitioner (objective) pain score	Severe pain	Mild pain
Reason for variance – using pain behaviours	**'Disabling, stops normal activities'**. Unable to walk unaided, cannot concentrate on verbal responses and has marked physiological changes in heart rate, respiratory rate and looks in severe pain	**'Few problems, can do most things'**. Able to walk, talk and illustrates only mild discomfort during the triage event

The contrasting cases illustrate the importance of applying both patient and triage practitioner pain scores and refutes the notion that the objective score is there to undermine or downplay what the patient's assessment of their pain is.

Analgesia at triage

There are significant benefits to the administration of effective analgesia at the outset of the patient's journey, which include:

- Pain management at the point of entry
- Patients have rapid access to analgesia
- Pain managed at the earliest opportunity
- Reduction in pain with early, effective analgesia
- Reduced stress and anxiety, improving communication
- Reprioritisation may be possible

Ensuring that triage practitioners have the knowledge, skill and professional indemnity to make decisions on the safe administration of effective analgesia is a valuable aspect of the triage assessment. It is important to recognise that asking patients about their level of pain during the triage event implies there will be some action to improve their pain.

Professional legislation is already in place in many major health economies to facilitate drug administration by triage practitioners, usually from a designated list of analgesics and indicated patient pain levels. The use of professional and legal frameworks such as standing orders or patient group directions (PGDs) provides a strong basis for patient safety. However, it needs to be acknowledged that not all triage practitioners are afforded the same professional scope of practice. In health economies yet to comprehend the benefits of drug administration by triage practitioners, there is a need to provide clear pathways of care ensuring a clinician prescribes timely and effective analgesia.

Summary

There is significant patient benefit when triage practitioners are trained to effectively assess pain, using a reliable and reproducible pain assessment tool that considers both patient and practitioner pain scoring. Combined with rapid administration of effective analgesia, at the outset of the patient's journey, this ensures that pain is managed at the earliest opportunity.

CHAPTER 5

Streaming with the Manchester Triage System

The Manchester Triage System (MTS) is designed to be a robust, auditable risk management tool that identifies the clinical priority of individual patients. Interestingly, the process of the MTS and the outcome of the triage consultation can also be used to allocate patients to specific areas of a service. The idea that all patients can be directed within a department or to other services that best meet the patient's needs, is known as **streaming**.

Streaming post triage event

Often the triage event includes more than the assessment and prioritisation of patients. In addition to being asked to prioritise patients and deliver basic first aid, triage practitioners may also be expected to do the following:

- Triage patients to GP appointments, pharmacy services or self-care
- Initiate agreed patient pathways to facilitate direct referral to in-patient specialties
- Initiate agreed patient pathways to facilitate scheduled appointments for out-patient specialties

In many cases these activities require a high level of decision making, with associated training needs in the assessment of patients, and a detailed understanding of any agreed referral processes. The pressure on triage practitioners to identify safe and appropriate allocation of services for patients can be stressful, however the benefits are that patients often avoid unnecessary delay when directed to alternative services/specialties from triage.

Streaming using the presentation–priority matrix

The idea of the inappropriate patient has largely been replaced by the concept of inappropriate care delivery and patient choice. Multiple entry gates to urgent and emergency care, and the development of an 'emergency care village', have become a reality in many healthcare systems.

It became clear when reviewing the second edition of *Emergency Triage* that the outcome of the prioritisation process could be captured to inform decisions about the most appropriate disposition of the patient. The combination of the selected presentation flowchart and allocated priority could be mapped to a whole range of care provision. For example, a patient presenting with a limb problem allocated to green/priority 4 is best streamed to a minor injuries/urgent treatment centre, while a patient with cardiac chest pain allocated to the orange/priority 2 is best managed in the resuscitation room. The mapping process was further refined to produce the MTS presentation–priority matrix (PPM) with accompanying detailed instructions for best results.

The PPM process

The current iteration of the PPM has been designed using this edition of *Emergency Triage*. The MTS consists of 54 patient presentations, most with five priorities, making a total of 266 presentation–priority combinations. A structured mapping process can be undertaken, by any service, to consider and identify appropriate dispositions for each of the 266 priority presentations. The process involves reviewing each of the triage outcomes and deciding, at a local level, the most appropriate stream/disposition for that patient presentation and assigned priority.

The dispositions available will be subject to local urgent and emergency care provision, which will differ from region to region and country to country. For example, the lack of an emergency eye unit will change where patients with eye problems are managed. An identified lack of a service may stimulate debate with local commissioners to provide a more appropriate service for patients.

Some health economies have embraced the 'emergency village' concept and have developed multiple streams for patient populations. The list of possible streams and dispositions (Table 5.1) is an example of the varied choices that could apply to many services. It is, however, acknowledged that some healthcare systems/countries have limited streams, existing within the emergency department alone, but the PPM will still be an equally effective tool in these circumstances.

Table 5.1 Examples of urgent and emergency care streams/dispositions

Disposition code	Disposition description
R	Resus room – emergency department
Ma	Majors area – emergency department
Mi	Minors area
UTC	Urgent treatment centre (aligns best with traditional minors area)
SDEC	Same day emergency care
MAU/SAU/PAU	Assessment units (medical (MAU), surgical (SAU), paediatric (PAU), etc.)
GP	General practitioner service based in urgent/emergency care – urgent or scheduled appointment
PC	Primary care scheduled appointment
PSY	Psychiatric assessment/crisis team
DENT	Dental appointment
EYE	Eye hospital or clinic
SHC	Sexual health clinic
PHA	Pharmacy
SC	Self-care

Engaging key stakeholders

It will be necessary to identify who needs to complete the mapping exercise and contribute to the consensus. In the event patients will be directed across a range of services it is useful to engage different providers and professional groups to provide a balanced view of how patients should be streamed.

Stakeholders are often identified from the list of dispositions. Carefully consider individuals with a vested interest in the outcome of the PPM, for example those who hold clinical accountability such as clinical directors, consultants and senior nurse managers as well as triage practitioners who will be using the tool.

The first task of the stakeholder team is to establish the list of streams/dispositions that patients can be directed to. These dispositions could be within the emergency department and in units and specialties across the wider organisation and local community. Once a final list has been identified and agreed, it is used by the stakeholders to complete the matrix. Stakeholders must be made aware that only the agreed list should be used when completing the PPM table, to prevent individuals from adding new dispositions to the process. Each organisation completing a PPM will produce a unique map that is tailored to the streams/services available to them.

How to complete the PPM

Obtain a copy of the latest edition or update of *Emergency Triage*. The PPM must be completed as an open book exercise with each stakeholder basing their streaming decisions on the same methodology that the triage practitioners will be using for the final matrix.

Provide each stakeholder with:

- Access to the latest version of presentation flowcharts
- A copy of the blank matrix
- The agreed list of streams/dispositions

Identified stakeholders will independently review each presentation flowchart, priority by priority, starting at the top of each chart and working down (red to blue). Whilst reviewing a chart, they decide for each of the priorities which disposition they feel is most appropriate for the patient. For example, a red outcome in nearly all charts would result in a PPM disposition of 'resus', however a yellow outcome in one presentation flowchart may result in a different disposition than in another chart because of the discriminators present. Black boxes indicate that the MTS chart chosen does not contain that priority.

Within a given timeframe each of the stakeholders completes the matrix with their decisions and returns to the nominated person to collate all the responses.

Collating the results

Once all stakeholders have completed the template, all the forms require collating by the nominated person and reviewing to identify where there is agreement and where dispositions may differ. Where there is a majority agreement the most frequently chosen disposition will be agreed as the PPM outcome for that chart and priority. If there is more than one service mapped that may be appropriate for a particular chart and priority, it is acceptable to place more than one disposition in the final matrix.

The collated results in Table 5.2 illustrate a complete consensus in red priority for a head injury presentation. However, in the green priority, the 10 stakeholders have chosen three different dispositions, but consensus could be met as 6/10 agree on primary care as the disposition.

Table 5.2 Example of collated results

Chart	Priority	Stream/disposition	Stakeholders (*N* = 10)
Head injury	Red	Resus	10
Head injury	Green	Primary care	6
Head injury	Green	Minors area	2
Head injury	Green	Self-care	2

The review process

Where no clear decision can be reached, or in cases where a variety of streams/dispositions are identified, each one should be added to the matrix and this subset returned to stakeholders asking them to list them in order of their most popular choice. The results of this iteration are again reviewed, and the process continues until there is a consensus and the disposition can be added to the final matrix. It will be down to the stakeholder team to decide what constitutes a majority decision, but it is essential that stakeholders working to develop the matrix finally reach a consensus decision.

The first time the PPM is developed the process of initial review and subsequent revision may take some time. However, once a consensus is agreed for each chart and priority, the result is an agreed matrix that best meets the service provision, and evaluation of the utility of the matrix can begin.

Quick reference on how to complete the PPM

- Establish the list of dispositions to which patients can be directed (see Table 5.1)
- Provide each stakeholder with a blank matrix and a copy of the 4th edition of *Emergency Triage*; this is strictly an open book exercise to ensure each stakeholder bases their decisions on the same methodology as the triage practitioners
- Individual stakeholders use a reductionist approach (start at red/priority 1 and work down to blue/priority 5) to consider for each of the presentation charts which disposition is appropriate for the patient in a particular priority, for example:
  - Asthma — priority 1 — inadequate breathing = resuscitation room
  - Dental problems — priority 4 — recent mild pain = dental service
  - Limb problem — priority 3 — moderate pain = minor treatment area
- There may be certain points in the matrix where stakeholders are unsure of a particular disposition. In those instances the boxes should be left blank to avoid skewing the consensus
- All completed matrices should be collated; where consensus is not reached further iteration is required until a clear map of agreed dispositions is produced

A completed PPM

Table 5.3 offers an example of how a completed matrix may look and has been populated to illustrate a comprehensive range of dispositions that could feasibly be used within an urgent and emergency care service. The streams, derived from consensus, form the basis of dispositions within the PPM. Triage practitioners use the matrix at the end of each triage consultation to identify the agreed stream for that patient. The triage practitioner may on occasion need to exercise judgement as to which is the most appropriate stream, as the decision may also be influenced by the availability of services across 24 hours, current pressures on the service and in some circumstances patient choice.

Periodic evaluation

Evaluation of the PPM requires periodic review to ensure all streams/dispositions remain appropriate for each chart and priority in response to patient outcomes. Also, as new services become available, or change, they can be added or indeed removed from the matrix to ensure patients are provided with the most appropriate care.

Table 5.3 MTS *Emergency Triage* 4th edition PPM

	1	2	3	4	5
Abdominal pain in adults	**R**	Ma	SAU/Ma^{P}	GP/PC	GP/PC
Abdominal pain in children	**R**	R/Ma	PAU/Ma	GP/PC	GP/PC
Abscesses and local infections	**R**	Ma	Mi	GP/PC	GP/PC
Abuse and neglect	**R**	R	Ma	PAU	
Allergy	**R**	R	Ma^{P}	GP/PC	GP/PC
Apparently drunk	**R**	R/Ma	Ma	Mi	SC
Assault	**R**	R	Ma	Mi	SC
Asthma	**R**	R	Ma	GP/PC	GP/PC
Back pain	**R**	Ma	Mi^{P}	GP/PC	PC/PHA
Behaving strangely	**R**	Ma	Mi/PSY	Mi/PSY	PC
Bites and stings	**R**	R	Mi^{P}	GP/PC	GP/PC
Burns and scalds	**R**	R	Ma	Mi/UTC	PHA/SC
Chemical exposure	**R**	R	Ma	UTC	PC
Chest pain	**R**	R	Ma	SDEC	PC
Collapse	**R**	R	Ma	GP/PC	GP/PC
Crying baby	**R**	R	Ma/PAU	GP/PC	GP/PC
Dental problems	**R**	Ma	Mi	DENT	DENT
Diabetes	**R**	R/Ma	Ma/MAU	GP/PC	GP/PC
Diarrhoea and vomiting in adults	**R**	R	Ma^{P}	PC	SC
Diarrhoea and vomiting in children	**R**	R	Ma^{P}	PC	SC
Ear problems	**R**	Ma	Ma^{P}	PC	SC
Eye problems	**Ma**	Ma/EYE	Mi/EYE	Mi	PC
Facial problems	**R**	R/Ma	Ma	Mi	PC
Falls	**R**	R/Ma	Ma	Mi	PC
Fits	**R**	R	Ma	Mi	PC
Foreign body	**R**	R/Ma	Mi	Mi	PC
GI bleeding	**R**	R	SAU/Ma	GP/PC	GP/PC
Head injury	**R**	R	Ma	Mi	SC
Headache	**R**	R	SDEC	Mi	PC
Irritable child	**R**	R	Ma^{P}	GP/PC	GP/PC
Limb problems	**R**	R/Ma	Ma	Mi	PC
Limping child	**R**	R/Ma	PAU	UTC	PC

(*Continued*)

Table 5.3 *(Continued)*

	1	2	3	4	5
Major trauma	**R**	R	Ma		
Mental illness	**R**	Ma	PSY	PSY	PC
Neck pain	**R**	Ma	Mi^{P}	PC	SC
Overdose and poisoning	**R**	R/Ma	Mi^{P}	PC	SC
Palpitations	**R**	R	Ma	GP/PC	GP/PC
Pregnancy	**R**	R	Ma^{P+}	GP/PC	GP/PC
PV bleeding	**R**	R/Ma	Ma^{P+}	GP/PC	GP/PC
Rashes	**R**	R	Mi^{P}	PC	SC
Self-harm	**R**	R	Mi/PSY	Mi/PSY	
Sexually acquired infection	**R**	R/Ma	SHC	SHC	PHA/SC
Shortness of breath in adults	**R**	R	Ma	GP/PC	GP/PC
Shortness of breath in children	**R**	R	Ma	GP/PC	GP/PC
Sore throat	**R**	Ma	Mi	PC	SC
Testicular pain	**R**	Ma	Mi	Mi	GP/PC
Torso injury	**R**	R	Mi	Mi	PC
Unwell adult	**R**	R	Ma^{P}	GP/PC	GP/PC
Unwell baby up to 12 months	**R**	R	PAU	GP/PC	GP/PC
Unwell child	**R**	R	Ma^{P}	GP/PC	GP/PC
Unwell newborn up to 28 days	**R**	R	Ma	PAU	PC
Urinary problems	**R**	Ma	Ma^{P}	GP/PC	GP/PC
Worried parent	**R**	R	Ma^{P}	GP/PC	GP/PC
Wounds	**R**	R/Ma	Mi	Mi	SC

Practical advantages of the PPM

- Benefit to triage practitioners – not spending time trying to work out where the patient should be placed within the service
- Inexperienced triage practitioners are relieved of the stress of having to make these higher level decisions
- Patients can be rapidly allocated to the agreed stream without triage practitioners having to seek permission or check their decision is acceptable with the area coordinator
- Removes personal choice and preferences around patient disposition, as each triage outcome is decided by consulting the matrix which is the departmental agreement for disposition
- Provides consistency as to where patients are streamed that is not based on how busy the service is, but what disposition best serves that patient's needs
- Offers a patient safety benefit when using the PPM as patients are not only allocated to the most appropriate area but they will also be received by the most appropriate clinicians

Streams of care

The development of a strong and locally tailored PPM can be used to drive timely and effective patient care in systems that have adopted streaming. Presentation–priority combinations (e.g. wounds–green, chest pain–orange) may be appropriate to specific streams, minor injuries and resuscitation in the examples given. Streaming is a similar concept to 'fast tracking', where particular groups of patients (usually those with relatively minor injuries and illnesses) are identified and seen by dedicated staff to improve patient flow.

Many streams are professionally led rather than patient led. It is feasible to provide a number of services within a single area such as an 'urgent treatment centre' which approximately maps onto the traditional 'minors area' of many emergency departments. There is obvious scope for many of these urgent and emergency care services to coalesce within an 'emergency care village' that also offers out-of-hours primary care provision and can not only relieve the burden of care in emergency departments but also offer appropriate patient choice.

The psychiatric disposition will be provided differently throughout the world and may include psychiatry and psychiatric nursing. Many urgent and emergency care services have emergency psychiatric nursing teams, and some are developing psychiatric assessment unit functions to expedite the management of this patient group.

Emergency dental service and eye emergency clinic dispositions also depend on local provision. The sexual health clinic disposition will again depend on location and opening times of local provision, although the specialist nature of the care delivered will dictate that most patients not requiring immediate or very urgent care are redirected. Other dispositions may be available locally and should be used where appropriate; however, the decision will also depend on opening times and the location of any such facilities and will often result in more than one disposition against a priority where services are not available 24/7.

Additional prompts in the PPM (^{P} and +)

The PPM can be used to indicate a number of extra prompts to triage practitioners as they check for the appropriate stream for a particular patient presentation and priority.

One such example is the selection of the moderate pain discriminator. In Table 5.3 numerous boxes contain a disposition with a 'P' symbol added, e.g. Ma^{P}/Mi^{P}.

When the symbol is noted this alerts the practitioner that following accurate assessment of pain using the MTS pain ruler, a patient who remains in yellow/priority 3 on this discriminator **alone** should be offered adequate analgesia. They should then be streamed to the disposition in the green/priority 4 box.

Another example is the use of a '+' symbol, whereby specific instructions can be prompted. Figure 5.1 is an example illustrating how extra actions related to specific presentations and priorities can work.

Chart	Discriminator	Action	Disposition
Abdominal pain in adults	Possibly pregnant	A patient who remains in yellow/priority 3 on this discriminator **alone** should be requested to provide a urine sample for pregnancy testing	Pregnancy test negative: refer GP/PC Pregnancy test positive: remain in Ma/refer SAU

Figure 5.1 Prompting extra actions

Highlighting additional patient pathways

There are often certain groups of patients with a pre-diagnosis, for example cardiac pain or fractured neck of femur, that may be subject to additional care pathways. The PPM can be used to highlight the use of a pathway to the triage practitioner who can initiate that protocol once triage is completed (see related symbol in Table 5.3). The value of highlighting where an additional pathway should be commenced means that patient management can be expedited according to the protocol without manipulating a priority, skewing the case mix or rendering audit unreliable.

Triage accuracy is key

The PPM can only be effective when based on accurate triage decision making. Rushed, inaccurate and unsafe triage decisions could result in patients being streamed to the wrong disposition.

CHAPTER **6**

Special considerations and patient populations

Introduction

There is a difference between absolute clinical priority, as defined using the Manchester Triage System (MTS), and relative priority within and between triage categories. In overview, the process of triage is quite simple in that patients are assigned to a triage category and then managed in order of priority and time of attendance. However, there are many other factors apart from clinical priority that may influence how the patient is handled within urgent and emergency care. This chapter outlines these factors and discusses their importance. Clinical priority and the findings that determine it are clearly very important, but failure to recognise other factors can be detrimental to both departmental function and quality of care for individual patients.

Departmental factors

Any service dealing with emergencies may at times be overwhelmed by the influx of patients. Sometimes, it only takes one seriously ill patient, or an absent member of staff, to produce a standstill and units need to develop means of coping with this situation. An accurate triage assessment is an essential first step in good departmental management.

Both the workload and the staffing of the service will vary according to the time of day. Frequently, during the night there is reduced clinical staffing. This may cause increased waiting times and difficulties in the waiting room, particularly if there are patients who are aggressive or under the influence of alcohol.

Role of the triage practitioner

The triage practitioner's main role is the accurate prioritisation of patients, and this must be the prime objective. They need to become accomplished at rapid assessment; this involves quick decision making and suitable delegation of tasks.

In small units, the triage practitioner will see all patients coming into the service. In others, there may be separate practitioners dealing with patients who arrive on foot or by ambulance. The mode of arrival of the patient does not always correlate with the seriousness of the presenting problem. Patients with trivial complaints may call the emergency services and patients with a myocardial infarction may arrive by car. Therefore, there must be close liaison between triage and clinical areas to ensure that patients are placed in the appropriate location.

Rapid influxes of patients may require the triage practitioner to seek assistance from other members of staff. The triage process is integral to the clinical management of most urgent and emergency care services.

Patient information

The triage practitioner is the first clinical contact for the patient, and taking the patient through the illness and probable course of their patient journey can alleviate distress and anxiety. Patients appreciate knowing the waiting time, the probable time spent in the department, whether any investigations may be ordered and possible treatment. This information can be provided quickly regarding the most common conditions.

Health promotion

The triage practitioner, time permitting, can usefully act as a health promoter. The patient is usually interested in receiving healthcare advice. Sometimes brief advice about relevant topics, for example self-medication, cycle helmets and smoking cessation, may be appropriate. It is helpful to provide patient information leaflets to reinforce the health discussion as the patient may be in pain, distracted or unreceptive at the time.

Specific patient populations

There are several issues regarding particular groups of patients that may affect their management in addition to their clinical priority. A range of patient populations, by no means exhaustive, are discussed here in more detail with specific issues highlighted for each.

Children

Children may need specific consideration, especially in emergency departments without separate paediatric facilities. They are almost always accompanied by someone else (usually a parent, but teachers, relatives or carers may also be present), as well as siblings and friends who, although well, need entertainment. Young children have particularly short attention spans and get bored, frightened and tired very easily. They may become distressed and agitated because of communication and understanding difficulties, and this makes any subsequent treatment and management more difficult.

Children who can be distracted by a play specialist, or in a separate waiting room with age-specific facilities, probably do not need any particular consideration other than frequent reassessment. It is helpful if child-friendly food and drink (e.g. snacks and drinks in cartons, bottles, etc.) is available, provided the carer of any child who may need a general anaesthetic or sedation is aware of the need to keep the child nil by mouth.

It may be worthwhile having a policy for children who present late in the evening or at night; however, this will be in the form of a patient pathway and not manipulation of the triage priority. The child who is very tired may prove impossible to examine and treat, so a relatively early examination can be considered.

Frail elderly patients

As the proportion of elderly people across the world is increasing, many patients attending urgent and emergency care services will be classed as elderly and may also be frail. A person who is normally able to cope well with familiar surroundings may become confused and disorientated in the chaotic and noisy environment common in urgent and emergency care. These issues may be further compounded for this group of patients by difficulties with vision, hearing and also cognitive impairment, such as dementia, which may result in them providing limited or inaccurate information.

Delerium is a serious consequence for elderly frail patients and is characterised by acute confusion and fluctuating cognition. Delerium is prevalent in acute care settings, including emergency departments, especially in patients over the age of 65 years and is associated with a significant increase in mortality and morbidity in this group. Rapidly identifying and managing delirium is critical for improved patient care and the use of effective screening tools, alongside staff education, is key.

Relative immobility can cause increased discomfort in the waiting room and may cause difficulty for the patient in reaching the toilet or going for refreshments. The elderly are prone to pressure damage to tissues, which can develop after just thirty minutes on a hospital trolley. They may have problems with continence which, if not anticipated, may lead to embarrassment and further risk of tissue damage. Practitioners should be aware of these issues and consider the relative needs of this group of patients. Where further assessment and management is delayed, they need frequent nursing attention. In many services frailty scores are recorded on arrival to highlight the most vulnerable patients invoking pathways of care to expedite patient management and ensure they are cared for in a suitable environment.

Patients with physical disability or learning difficulties

Apart from the extremes of age, there will be patients who have particular difficulties. These include those with special needs, poor sight, poor hearing, etc. People who can cope quite well in the community under controlled circumstances may have great difficulties in the strange environment of the emergency department. Communication is particularly important, and it may be appropriate for such patients to be seen relatively quickly.

Patients with mental health problems

Previous editions of the MTS have consistently incorporated mental health flowcharts, recognising the importance of assessing this patient group. In 2021/2022 following a multiprofessional, international Delphi study, post publication updates were made to *Emergency Triage* (version 3.8) including the addition of 19 new discriminators (see Further reading).

These significant changes marked an important evolution of the MTS as for the first time there was equal parity of importance for both physical and mental health patient presentations. The additional discriminators included four red/priority 1 discriminators that established life-threatening emergencies that can and do occur with mental health presentations. Further very urgent, urgent and standard discriminators were added to a whole range of presentation flowcharts, and a fifth priority (blue) was added to all but one of the suite of mental health charts. The purpose of introducing the additional discriminators was to improve patient safety for mental health presentations when using the MTS at the point of entry to a service.

This group of patients is often subject to lengthy delays for referrals to psychiatric services, even when triaged to the highest of priorities. A busy and chaotic environment like urgent and emergency care is not conducive to these patients, often resulting in them becoming increasingly agitated and dysregulated. Careful consideration as to the most suitable and safe environment in which to place these patients is essential, alongside frequent assessments and monitoring of mood and behaviour for signs of deterioration that would require re-triage.

Abusive/aggressive patients

There are real challenges for busy triage practitioners when dealing with a full waiting room, with one or more patients (or more often relatives or friends of patients) constantly demanding attention. Although the guiding principle must be that these patients are not given priority, just because they shout louder, the distress they cause to others must be taken into consideration. An initial attempt to communicate departmental policy may be followed by a number of actions. The patient may be placed in an individual cubicle in order to minimise the disruption to the waiting room. Alternatively, such patients can be seen, treated and discharged rapidly for the benefit of others. If all else fails, the patient (or the patient's relatives) may be asked to leave, assisted, as necessary, by security or the police.

Patients under the influence of alcohol

These patients are difficult to assess because of the effect of alcohol on conscious level and pain perception. They need frequent reassessment to check that they are not deteriorating or developing a problem not immediately apparent at triage. Disruptive drunk patients can be managed similarly to the abusive/aggressive patients.

Patients requiring time critical medications

An increasing number of patients rely on time critical medications (TCM) and any visit, emergency or routine, to urgent and emergency care has the potential to significantly disrupt their medication schedule. Consideration of TCM must extend beyond obvious examples such as type 1 diabetes and should also encompass patients with Parkinson disease, epilepsy and indeed any patient where early or delayed administration of a scheduled dose of their medications may cause harm or result in suboptimal therapy or pharmacological effect. It is important to acknowledge that the majority of these patients are experts in managing their own health conditions and triage practitioners not only need to ask about TCM but actively listen to the patient and facilitate their requirements.

High frequency attendees

Most departments have patients who frequently attend that service, and it is undoubtedly tempting to place these patients in the non-urgent category without proper assessment. However, it is important to remember that this patient group can develop organic pathology, injure themselves or have a serious complication of a pre-existing illness. These patients, even those with predominantly social problems, are in fact more likely to develop illnesses or sustain injuries than the general population. Each attendance should be treated as a new visit and proper assessment should be undertaken; this avoids underestimation of possible serious causes for attendance.

Patients who reattend

There are occasions when patients return to the service, usually because their original presenting complaint has not resolved or they have developed a complication. Sometimes the patient's expectation of the natural progress of an injury or illness is unrealistic. The patient may also return having failed to wait for definitive treatment on a prior occasion. The patient should be allocated a triage category according to the symptoms presented at the time of triage, and not according to the original triage category. Some services may have policies recommending that such patients are reviewed by a senior clinician if available. It may also be appropriate to stream some of these patients to a scheduled clinic appointment for assessment by a GP or primary care clinician if the problem does not seem to warrant immediate treatment.

Patients referred to other agencies

Many departments find that their facilities are used by other teams for patient assessment. These patient visits are usually prearranged or they are accepted patients from primary care physicians for possible admission. Many have relatively high clinical priorities. These patients should be triaged in the same way as urgent and emergency care patients.

If the patient is triaged as red/priority 1 it would be usual for the emergency department team to initiate resuscitation, unless the referral team is present. The triage practitioner should inform the referral team of the patient's triage category to try and ensure the patient is treated with the correct degree of urgency. It may also be appropriate for the triage practitioner to ask departmental clinical staff to provide analgesia or initiate immediate investigations to expedite the patient's journey.

Some patients may have been brought in by the police (for instance under mental health legislation), by social services or by other professional services. Triage practitioners should be aware of the pressures on staff from other agencies and consider this when deciding on the management of such patients, but the triage priority would not change.

CHAPTER 7

The triage audit

Introduction

During their initial meeting in November 1994, the Manchester Triage Group clearly identified the need to establish a robust audit methodology. The reasons for this were that the Manchester Triage System (MTS) was designed to reduce unwarranted variations in the triage process, and this reduction could only be ensured by audit. Audit, in this context, is a quality management procedure; since triage is a fundamental cornerstone of clinical risk management, failure to ensure the quality of triage can have serious consequences.

Fortunately, the MTS methodology is eminently auditable. The presentation–discriminator–priority sequence (the process) by which individual triage practitioners arrive at their conclusions is easy for a trained MTS instructor to scrutinise and assess for accuracy.

In addition to the process of triage discussed, audit can also address other issues such as completeness of documentation and adherence with MTS terminology, in particular the correct application of discriminator definitions.

The audit process

At a basic level, the accuracy of individual triage practitioners underpins the whole quality agenda. Thus, the most robust triage audit continuously assesses practitioners for accuracy and is linked by reflective practice and, if necessary, additional training to improve performance.

The method outlined here is an audit of individual practitioner triage activity and is designed to audit the quality of decision making against the MTS standard, along with standards of record keeping and documentation:

- All triage practitioners are identified
- All episodes of triage are identified
- Episodes are all assigned to individual practitioners
- 2% of episodes per practitioner (minimum of 10 episodes) are randomly selected
- Episodes are assessed by a trained and current MTS instructor
- Completeness of episodes is expressed as a simple proportion, e.g. 9/10
- Accuracy of episodes is expressed as a simple proportion, e.g. 8/10
- Number of incomplete episodes is fed back to the triage practitioner
- Overall accuracy is fed back to the triage practitioner
- Any causes or trends of inaccurate triage identified are fed back to the triage practitioner

The audit method

Continuous audit, whilst time consuming, is an excellent means of assessing standards of triage activity and decision making across the whole team of triage practitioners.

In services first introducing the MTS, monthly audit is advised to establish confidence amongst practitioners using the system. This early scrutiny not only establishes accuracy and completeness of records but also starts to reveal the case mix of clinical activity, types of patient presentation and numbers of patients within each priority. Depending on how quickly accuracy reaches the requisite level, the frequency of audit may be reduced to 3–6 monthly thereafter.

An annual audit is a significant undertaking but even in large departments triaging 100 000 patients each year, the number audited is only 2000 cases per year or 160 per month. The criteria in Table 7.1 have been shown to capture the essential components of a safe and reproducible triage system.

Table 7.1 Audit criteria
Appropriate communication with the patient
Correct selection of the presentational flowchart
Appropriate observations recorded as per flowchart
Correct choice of highest order discriminator
Pain score recorded (subjective and objective)
Analgesia administered as per patient group direction (PGD) if required
Correct triage priority assigned (based on patient presentation and discriminator)
Correct presentation–priority matrix (PPM) assigned (based on patient presentation and discriminator)
Demonstration of the ability to navigate either a computerised triage system or manual system
Free text appropriate to patient presentation

Important note

MTS instructors – those experienced triage practitioners who have received additional training and support to audit the MTS – should be the only individuals who undertake this important function.

There are two important measures of the triage process that are obtained during each audit cycle: completeness and accuracy.

Completeness

An episode is complete if all the steps necessary to reach a safe and reproducible triage priority and documentation of the event have been undertaken. The method requires that the triage practitioner excludes all the discriminators in any higher priority. Thus, if very low SpO_2 appears as a discriminator in the chart selected, then the episode would be incomplete if no result was recorded. The most common error is failing to record a pain score. Therefore, both subjective and objective pain scores need to be mandatory fields, a requirement that is especially effective with computerised systems.

Accuracy

An episode is recorded as accurate if both the presentation and discriminator selected are appropriate. It is important to realise that there may be appropriate alternatives (indeed the system is designed to ensure that this can occur) but this is the reason why audit should be carried out by a trained MTS instructor with sufficient experience to make this judgement.

Audit targets

- 0% episodes incomplete
- 95% accuracy
- 95% agreement between auditors

Triage in practice

The triage audit will have a few additional effects on the triage process. It is not possible to carry out the audit without accurate triage notes and any deficiencies in record making will be highlighted. For instance, failure to record a pain score will mean that the auditor cannot be sure whether the triage priority assignment is correct. The result will then be marked as an incomplete episode; this encourages pain assessment to be undertaken and recorded. Similarly, failure to record required physiological measurements, such as temperature in the unwell child, will result in incomplete episodes. Feedback on a regular basis will improve the quality of these assessments, and experience has shown that this is an early 'win' from audit.

Minimum requirements for audit

- Whenever audit is undertaken by an MTS instructor the activity must be an open book exercise with access to the most up-to-date version of *Emergency Triage*
- MTS instructors work through the charts, using the same reductionist methodology, to assess the triage providers' decision making
- Using the MTS predetermined audit criteria (see Table 7.1), instructors check either 'Yes' or 'No' against each criterion. In some instance 'N/A' may apply (for example administration of analgesia if this scope of practice does not exist)
- The 10 audit criteria will be added to complete accuracy. The standard applied is that triage practitioners (both new and established) reach the audit targets detailed, thus proving competence

Establishing an audit cycle

To ensure consistency of approach between various auditors, 10% of episodes assessed are performed independently by a second trained MTS instructor and any differences moderated by discussion. Inter-rater reliability is an important feature of robust audit and should be established periodically within each audit cycle (Figure 7.1).

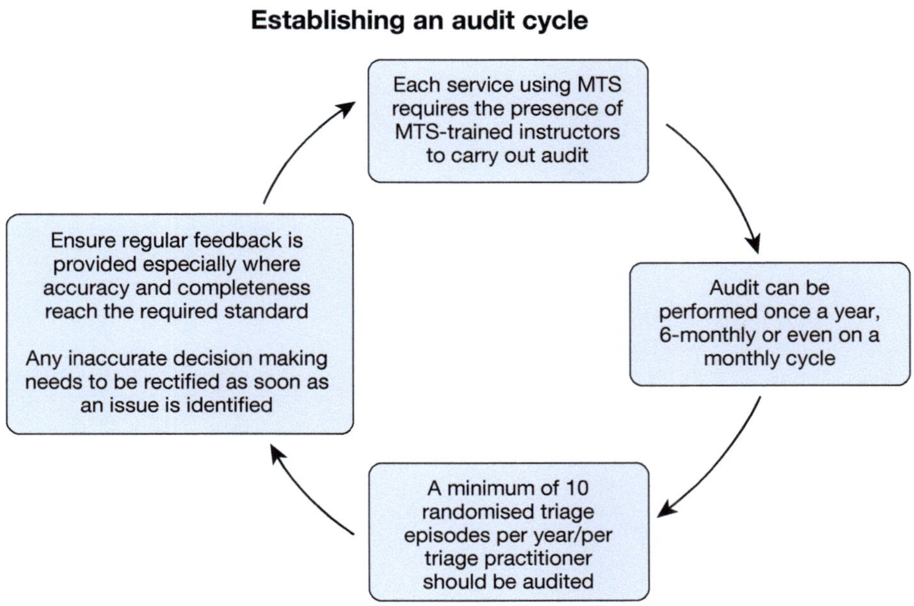

Figure 7.1 The audit cycle

National triage audit

In 2001 the MTS was introduced in Portugal as a national system in all public, private and military hospitals, having been trialled in a few hospitals prior to that time. The system is administered by the Portuguese Triage Group (Grupo Português de Triagem, GPT) who insisted from the outset that audit be an integral part of triage in all its areas of practice. All hospitals implementing the MTS are required to audit triage practitioners continuously and report the results to the GPT monthly. Twenty-five years of national data collection have shown consistently high levels of accuracy across Portugal and is an exemplar to all MTS users of the power of collecting this information.

Presentation flowchart index and how to use the charts

Presentation flowchart index

How to use the charts and notes

The charts are presented in alphabetical order for ease of use. Each chart has an accompanying facing page that offers an overview of the key uses and discriminators.

Related charts

For each chart the top of the facing page lists 'Related charts' where one or more charts may be listed. The listed charts are not meant to force the triage practitioner to look at multiple charts, as only one chart should be selected. The purpose of listing the related charts is a prompt that a more specific chart could be used, and the triage practitioner should therefore switch attention to the more specific chart.

Chart notes

These notes provide an overview of the presentation and attempt to briefly detail any possible pathologies, underlying conditions and age-related issues that should be considered when triaging with that chart.

The facing pages also contain a series of specific discriminators, and their definitions, that are most relevant to the chart. Adding the specific discriminators is meant for quick reference only and these pages are not a complete list of all the discriminators that appear in that chart. A full dictionary of every discriminator can be found on pages 179–189 and should be used as a constant source of information when triage practitioners are using the charts.

Presentation flowcharts

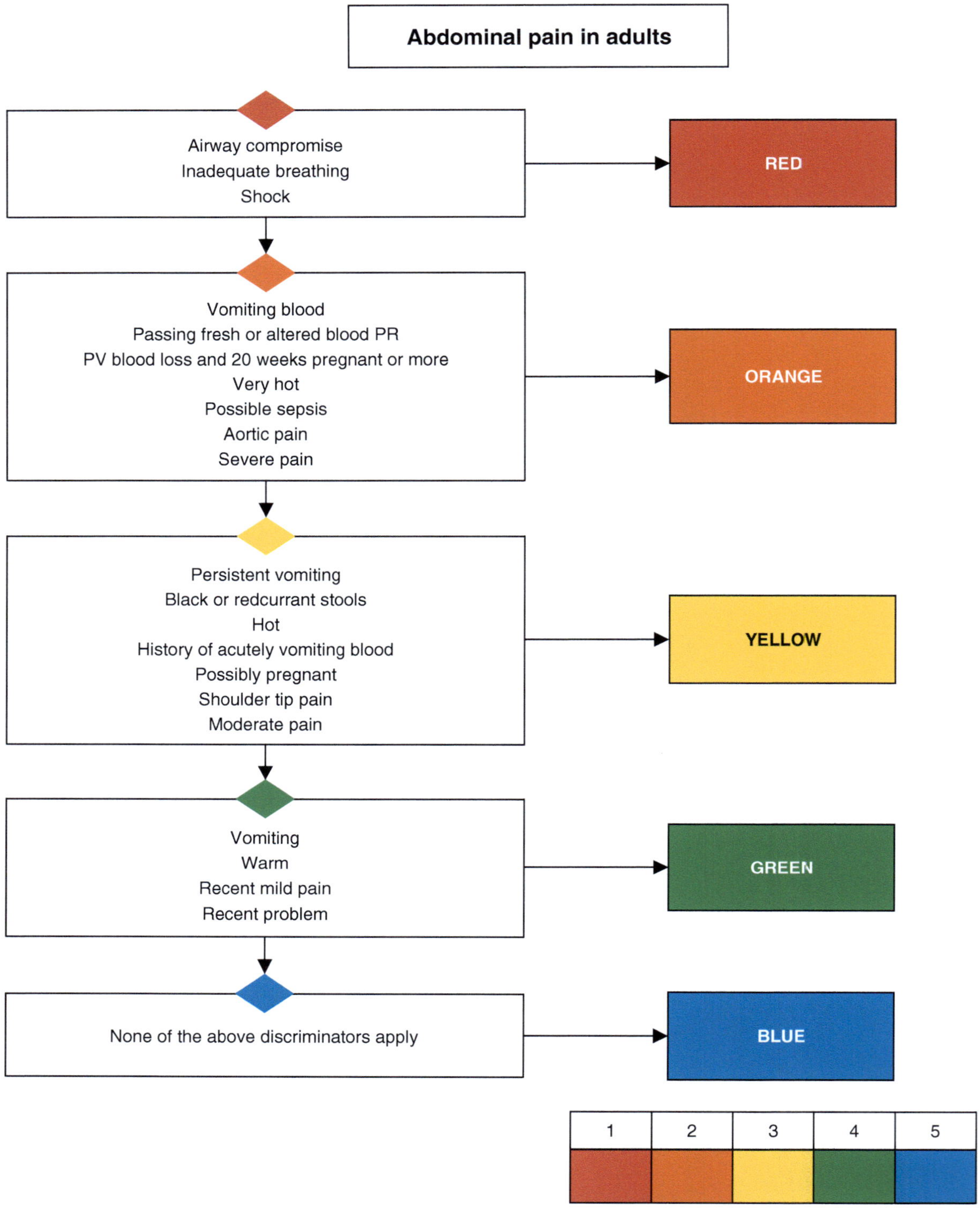
Abdominal pain in adults
Airway compromise
Inadequate breathing
Shock
RED
Vomiting blood
Passing fresh or altered blood PR
PV blood loss and 20 weeks pregnant or more
Very hot
Possible sepsis
Aortic pain
Severe pain
ORANGE
Persistent vomiting
Black or redcurrant stools
Hot
History of acutely vomiting blood
Possibly pregnant
Shoulder tip pain
Moderate pain
YELLOW
Vomiting
Warm
Recent mild pain
Recent problem
GREEN
None of the above discriminators apply
BLUE
1
2
3
4
5

Notes accompanying Abdominal pain in adults

Related charts	Chart notes
Diarrhoea and vomiting in adults GI bleeding Pregnancy	Abdominal pain is a common cause of presentation of surgical emergencies. A number of general discriminators are used including *Life threat* and *Pain*. Specific discriminators are included in the ORANGE and YELLOW categories to ensure that the more severe pathologies are appropriately triaged. In particular, discriminators are included to ensure that patients with moderate and severe GI bleeding and those with signs of retroperitoneal or diaphragmatic irritation are given sufficiently high categorisation

Relevant discriminators	Definition
Vomiting blood	Vomited blood may be fresh (bright or dark red) or coffee ground in appearance
Passing fresh or altered blood PR	In active massive GI bleeding, dark red blood will be passed PR. As GI transit time increases this becomes darker, eventually becoming melaena
PV blood loss and 20 weeks pregnant or more	Any loss of blood PV in a patient known to be beyond the 20th week of pregnancy
Aortic pain	The onset of symptoms is sudden and the leading symptom is severe abdominal or chest pain. The pain may be described as sharp, stabbing or ripping in character. Classically, aortic chest pain is felt around the sternum and then radiates to the shoulder blades; aortic abdominal pain is felt in the centre of the abdomen and radiates to the back. The pain may get better or even vanish and then recur elsewhere. Over time, pain may also be felt in the arms, neck, lower jaw, stomach or hips
Persistent vomiting	Vomiting that is continuous or that occurs without any respite between episodes
Black or redcurrant stools	Any blackness fulfils the criteria of black stool while a dark red stool, classically seen in intussusceptions, is redcurrant stool
History of acutely vomiting blood	Frank haematemesis, vomiting of altered blood (coffee ground) or of blood mixed in the vomit within the past 24 hours
Possibly pregnant	Any patient whose normal menstruation has failed to occur is possibly pregnant and any patient of childbearing age who is having unprotected sex should be considered to be potentially pregnant
Shoulder tip pain	Pain felt in the tip of the shoulder. This often indicates diaphragmatic irritation

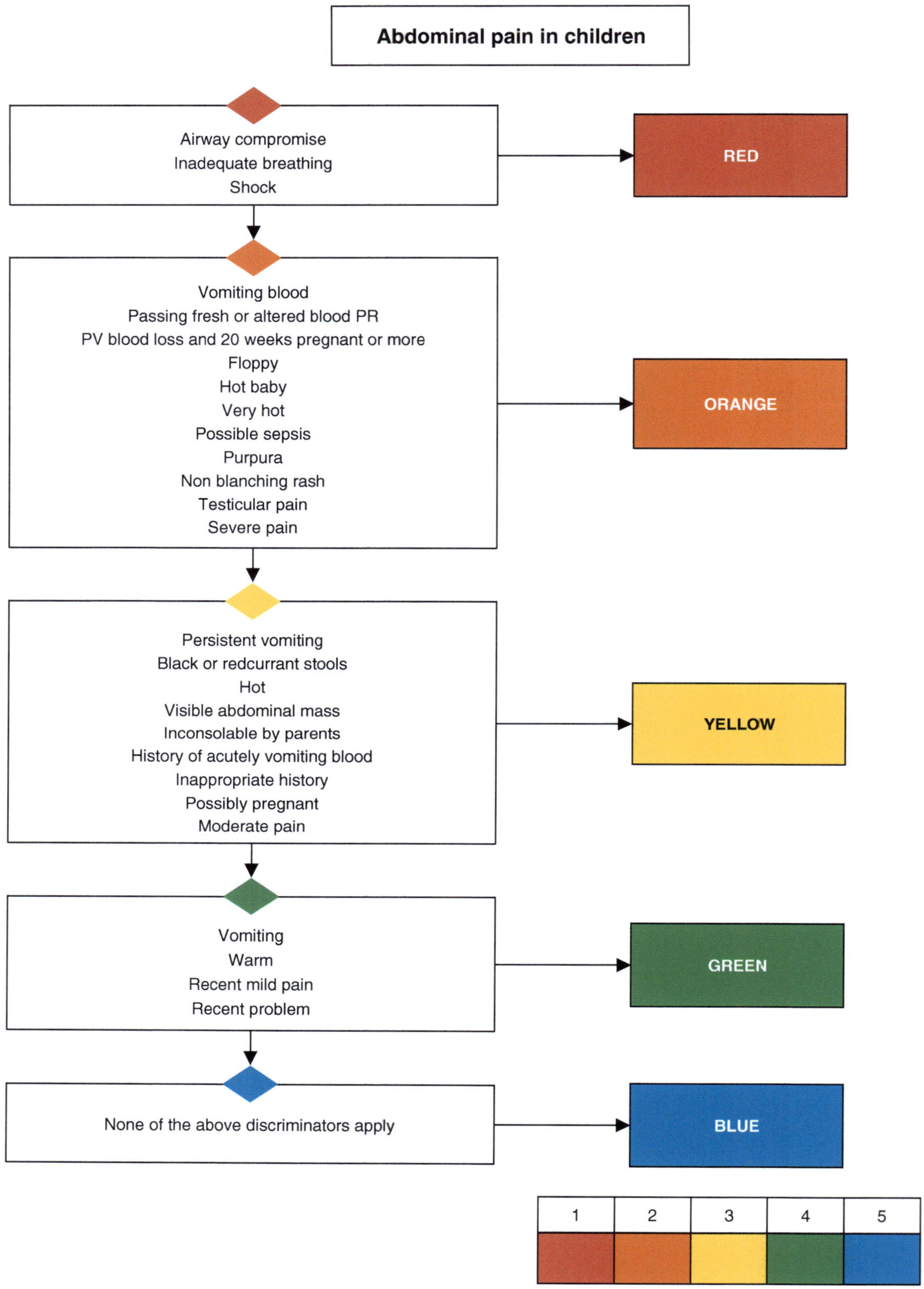
Abdominal pain in children
Airway compromise
Inadequate breathing
Shock
RED
Vomiting blood
Passing fresh or altered blood PR
PV blood loss and 20 weeks pregnant or more
Floppy
Hot baby
Very hot
Possible sepsis
Purpura
Non blanching rash
Testicular pain
Severe pain
ORANGE
Persistent vomiting
Black or redcurrant stools
Hot
Visible abdominal mass
Inconsolable by parents
History of acutely vomiting blood
Inappropriate history
Possibly pregnant
Moderate pain
YELLOW
Vomiting
Warm
Recent mild pain
Recent problem
GREEN
None of the above discriminators apply
BLUE
1
2
3
4
5

Notes accompanying Abdominal pain in children

Related charts	Chart notes
Diarrhoea and vomiting in children Unwell newborn	Children who present with abdominal pain may have a range of pathologies and this chart is designed to allow them to be accurately prioritised. A number of general discriminators are used including *Life threat* and *Pain*. Specific discriminators are included to ensure the children who are actively bleeding, and those who have the signs or symptoms of more severe pathologies such as intussusception, are seen urgently. If the patient is under 28 days, the Unwell newborn chart should be used

Relevant discriminators	Definition
Vomiting blood	Vomited blood may be fresh (bright or dark red) or coffee ground in appearance
Passing fresh or altered blood PR	In active massive GI bleeding, dark red blood will be passed PR. As GI transit time increases this becomes darker, eventually becoming melaena
PV blood loss and 20 weeks pregnant or more	Any loss of blood PV in a patient known to be beyond the 20th week of pregnancy
Testicular pain	Pain in the testicles
Persistent vomiting	Vomiting that is continuous or that occurs without any respite between episodes
Black or redcurrant stools	Any blackness fulfils the criteria of black stool while a dark red stool, classically seen in intussusceptions, is redcurrant stool
Visible abdominal mass	A mass in the abdomen that is visible to the naked eye
History of acutely vomiting blood	Frank haematemesis, vomiting of altered blood (coffee ground) or of blood mixed in the vomit within the past 24 hours
Possibly pregnant	Any patient whose normal menstruation has failed to occur is possibly pregnant and any patient, of childbearing age, who is having unprotected sex should be considered to be potentially pregnant

Abscesses and local infections

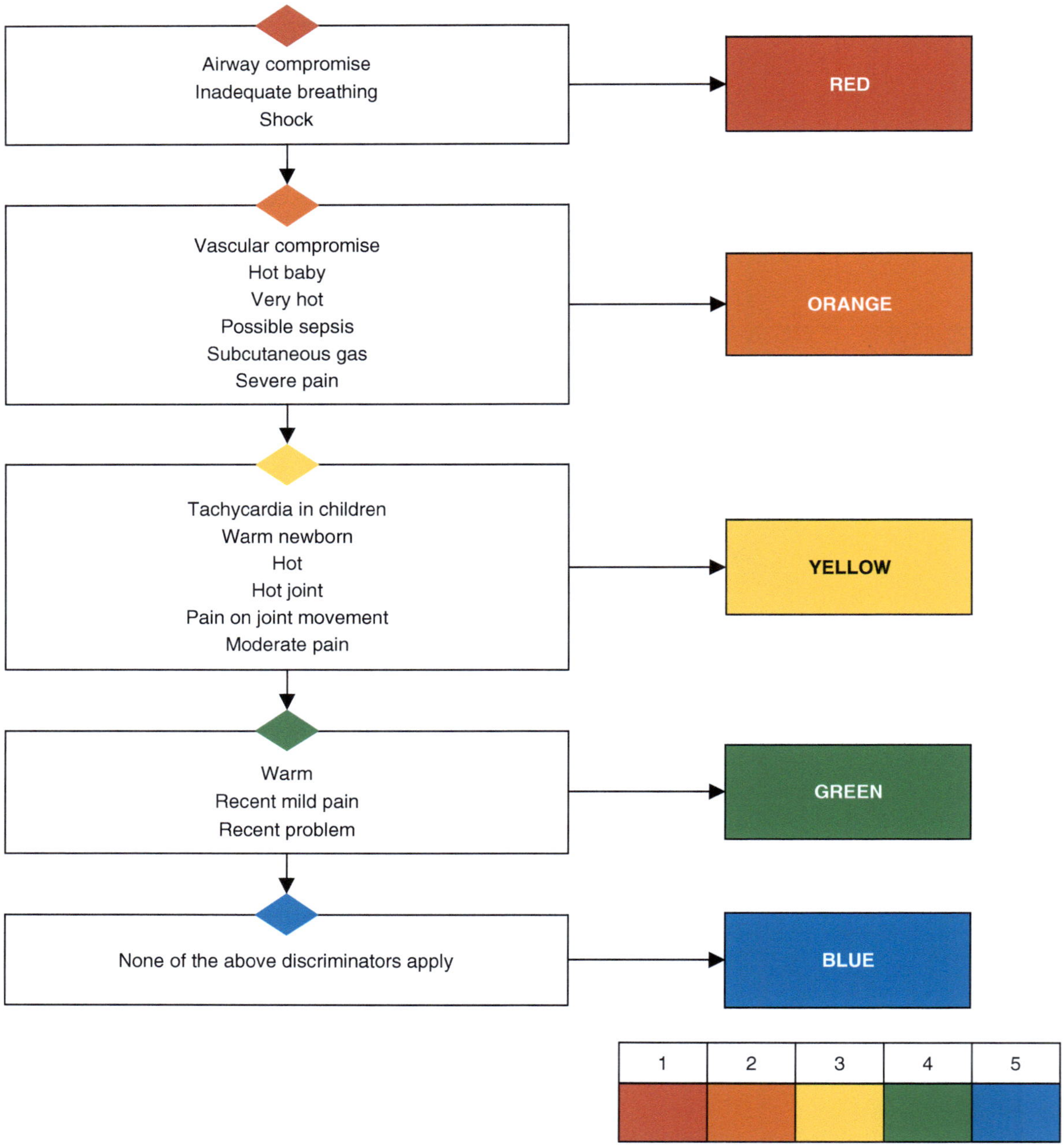

Notes accompanying Abscesses and local infections

Related charts	Chart notes
Bites and stings	This chart is designed to allow prioritisation of patients who present with a variety of obvious local infections and abscesses. Underlying conditions may vary from life-threatening orbital cellulitis to acneiform spots. A number of general discriminators are used including *Life threat, Pain* and *Temperature*. Specific discriminators have been included to allow identification of more urgent conditions such as gas gangrene and septic arthritis

Relevant discriminators	Definition
Vascular compromise	There will be a combination of pallor, coldness, altered sensation and pain with or without absent pulses distal to the injury
Possible sepsis	Suspected sepsis in patients who present with altered mental state, low blood pressure (systolic less than 100 mmHg) or raised respiratory rate (rate more than 22 breaths per minute) when using the qSOFA tool for assessment. Other sepsis screening tools may be used instead of qSOFA, and the relevant sepsis markers applied. In children, age-specific physiological tools should be used to determine if possibly septic
Subcutaneous gas	Gas under the skin can be detected by feeling for a 'crackling' on touch. There may be gas bubbles and a line of demarcation
Tachycardia in children	A child less than 1 year with a heart rate of 160 bpm or above ***OR*** a child 1 year or above with a heart rate of 140 bpm or above
Hot joint	Any warmth around a joint. Often accompanied by redness
Pain on joint movement	This can be pain on either active (patient) movement or passive (examiner) movement

Abuse and neglect

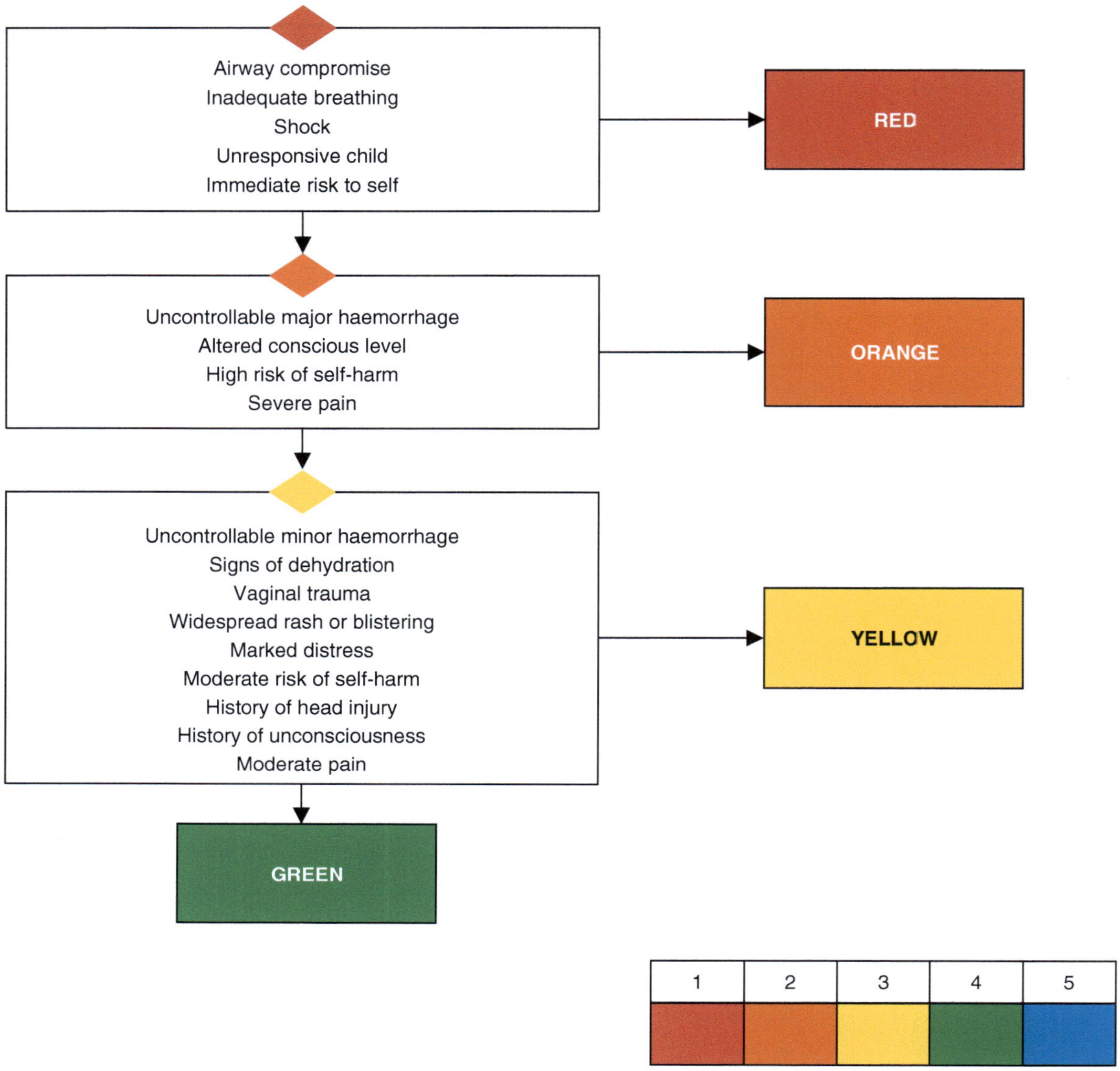

Notes accompanying Abuse and neglect

Related charts	Chart notes
None	This chart is designed to allow prioritisation of patients who present with signs of abuse or neglect. However, the presentation will be an obvious abuse or neglect issue, more often associated with a referral from a professional such as police, midwife, social worker, etc. The chart is not meant to be used because the triage practitioner has a suspicion of abuse and neglect and is not designed to triage illness or injury If the presentation is a physical illness or injury, it would be more appropriate to use a specific chart. A number of general discriminators are used including *Life threat, Conscious level* and *Pain*. Specific discriminators have been included to allow prioritisation of the most urgent cases

Relevant discriminators	Definition
Immediate risk to self	An initial view of the risk of harm to self can be formed by considering the patient's behaviour. Patients who are actively harming themselves and those who are threatening to harm themselves and who have the means to do so are at immediate risk
High risk of self-harm	An initial view of the risk of harm to self can be formed by considering the patient's behaviour. Patients who are threatening to harm themselves and who are actively seeking the means to do so are at high risk
Signs of dehydration	These include dry tongue, sunken eyes, decreased skin turgor and, in small babies, a sunken anterior fontanelle. Usually associated with a low urine output
Vaginal trauma	Any history or other evidence of direct trauma to the vagina
Marked distress	Patients who are markedly physically or emotionally upset
Moderate risk of self-harm	An initial view of the risk of harm to self can be formed by considering the patient's behaviour. Patients without a significant history of self-harm, who are not actively trying to harm themselves, but who profess the desire to harm themselves are at moderate risk
History of head injury	A history of a recent physically traumatic event involving the head. Usually this will be reported by the patient but if the patient has been unconscious this history should be sought from a reliable witness

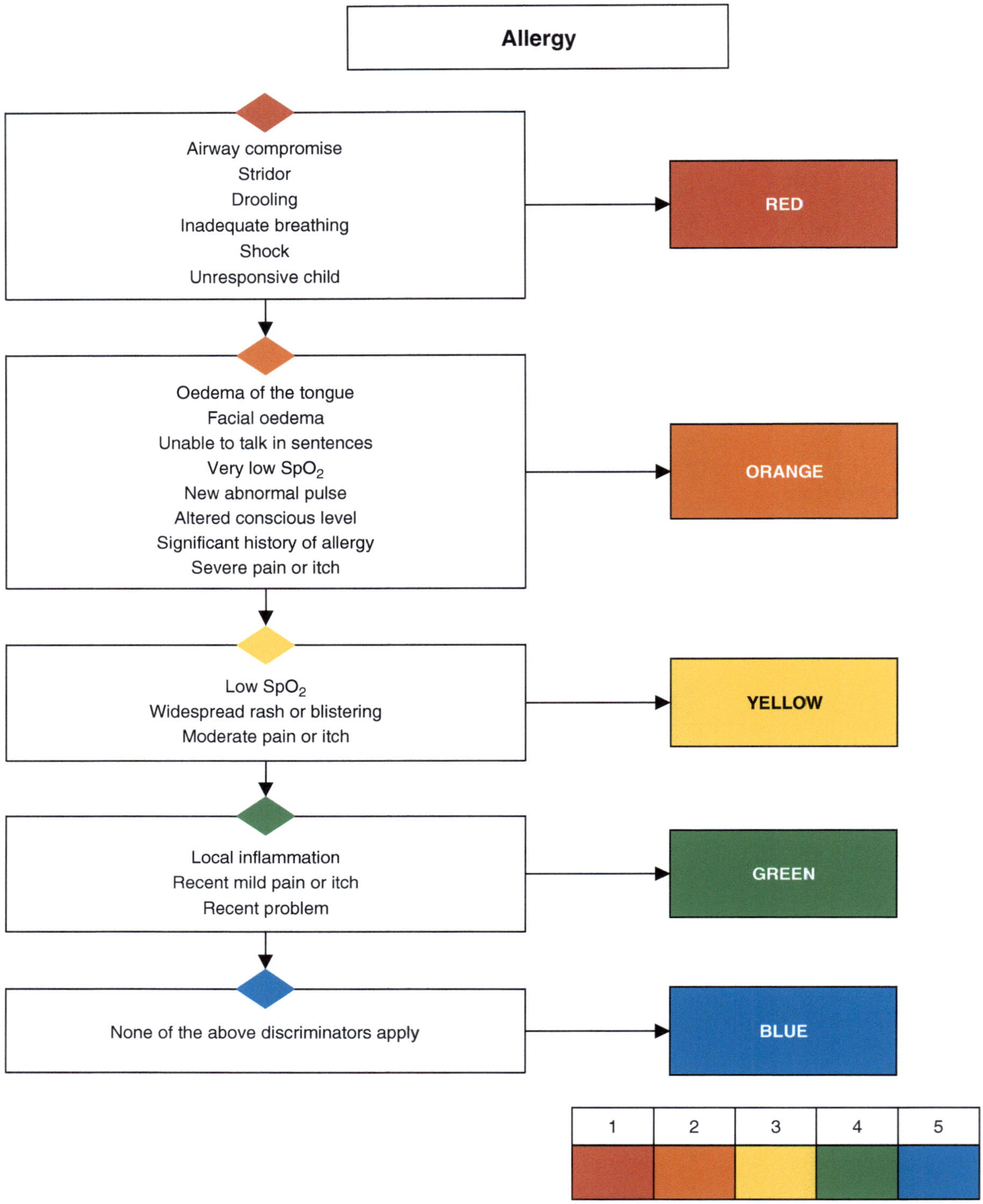
Allergy
Airway compromise
Stridor
Drooling
Inadequate breathing
Shock
Unresponsive child
RED
Oedema of the tongue
Facial oedema
Unable to talk in sentences
Very low SpO_2
New abnormal pulse
Altered conscious level
Significant history of allergy
Severe pain or itch
ORANGE
Low SpO_2
Widespread rash or blistering
Moderate pain or itch
YELLOW
Local inflammation
Recent mild pain or itch
Recent problem
GREEN
None of the above discriminators apply
BLUE
1
2
3
4
5

Notes accompanying Allergy

Related charts	Chart notes
Asthma Bites and stings Collapse Shortness of breath in adults Shortness of breath in children	This chart is designed to allow prioritisation of patients who present with symptoms and signs that may indicate allergy. Patients with allergic reactions range from those with life-threatening anaphylaxis to those with an itchy insect bite. A number of general discriminators are used including *Life threat, Conscious level* and *Pain*. Specific discriminators have been included to allow prioritisation of the most urgent conditions

Relevant discriminators	Definition
Stridor	This may be an inspiratory or expiratory noise, or both. Stridor is heard best on breathing with the mouth open
Drooling	Saliva running from the mouth as a result of being unable to swallow
Oedema of the tongue	Swelling of the tongue of any degree
Facial oedema	Diffuse swelling around the face, usually involving the lips
Unable to talk in sentences	Patients who are so breathless that they cannot complete relatively short sentences in one breath
Very low SpO_2	This is a saturation of less than 95% on O_2 therapy or less than 92% on air. The variation in risk according to skin colour necessitates the integration of pulse oximetry with other clinical and patient-reported data
Significant history of allergy	A known sensitivity with severe reaction (e.g. to nuts or bee sting) is significant
Low SpO_2	This is a saturation of less than 95% on air. The variation in risk according to skin colour necessitates the integration of pulse oximetry with other clinical and patient-reported data
Widespread rash or blistering	Any rash or blistering eruption covering more than 10% of the body surface area
Local inflammation	Local inflammation will involve pain, swelling and redness confined to a particular site or area

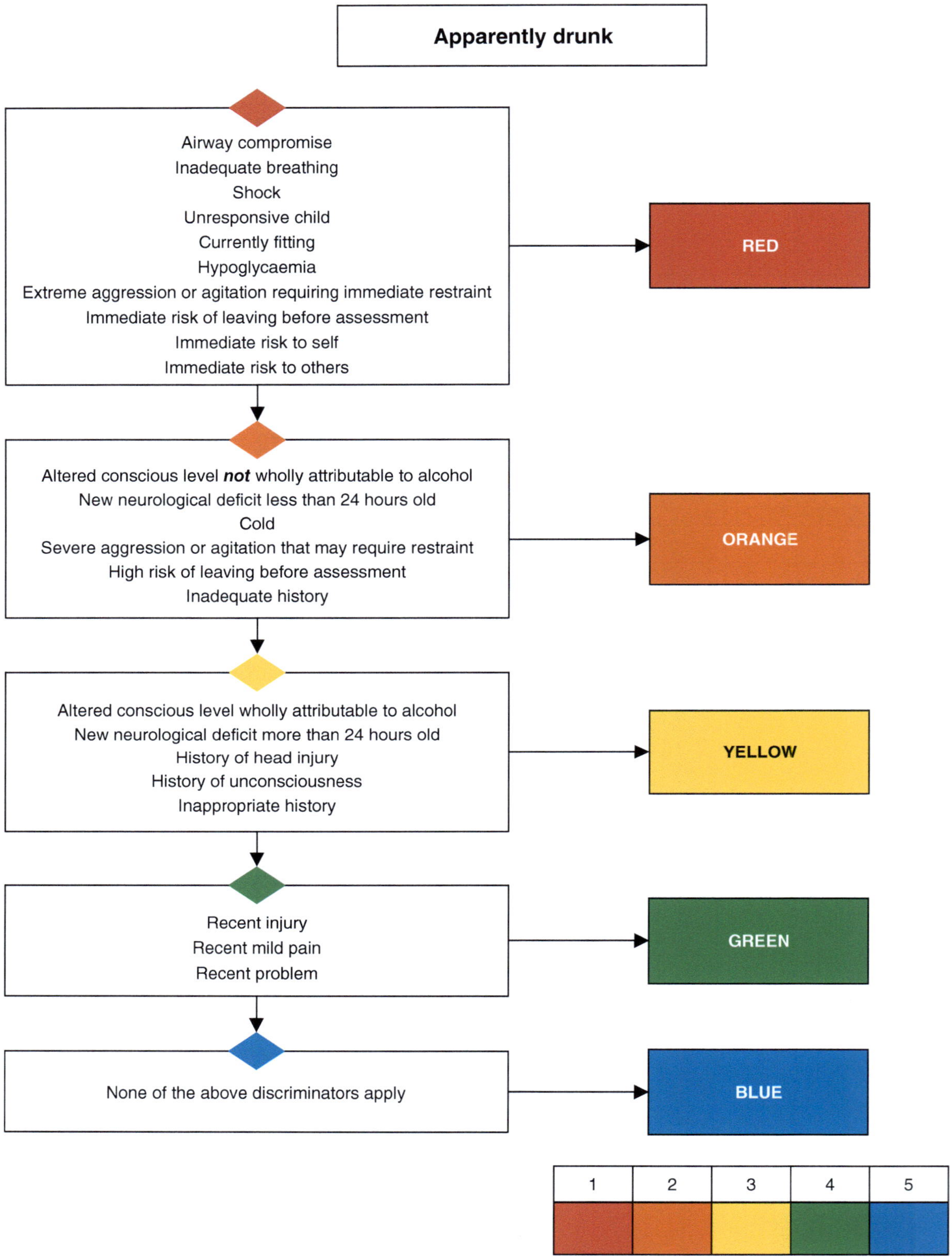
Apparently drunk
Airway compromise
Inadequate breathing
Shock
Unresponsive child
Currently fitting
Hypoglycaemia
Extreme aggression or agitation requiring immediate restraint
Immediate risk of leaving before assessment
Immediate risk to self
Immediate risk to others
RED
Altered conscious level *not* wholly attributable to alcohol
New neurological deficit less than 24 hours old
Cold
Severe aggression or agitation that may require restraint
High risk of leaving before assessment
Inadequate history
ORANGE
Altered conscious level wholly attributable to alcohol
New neurological deficit more than 24 hours old
History of head injury
History of unconsciousness
Inappropriate history
YELLOW
Recent injury
Recent mild pain
Recent problem
GREEN
None of the above discriminators apply
BLUE
1
2
3
4
5

Notes accompanying Apparently drunk

Related charts	Chart notes
Behaving strangely Collapse Head injury	A large number of patients attend for emergency treatment in an apparently drunken state. This chart implicitly recognises that not all these patients are drunk and is designed to ensure accurate identification and prioritisation of patients who are suffering from conditions which make them appear drunk, or from such severe drunkenness that their life is threatened. A number of general discriminators have been used including *Life threat, Conscious level in children* and *Blood glucose level*. Specific discriminators have been included to ensure that patients with an inadequate history of alcohol ingestion are seen rapidly and treated. If there is any doubt then the patient should be seen very urgently

Relevant discriminators	Definition
Hypoglycaemia	Glucose less than 3 mmol/l
Extreme aggression or agitation requiring immediate restraint	Aggression and agitation of such a degree that immediate restraint is required to manage the risk of harm to self or others
Immediate risk of leaving before assessment	Active, credible attempts to leave prior to assessment pose an immediate risk
Immediate risk to self	An initial view of the risk of harm to self can be formed by considering the patient's behaviour. Patients who are actively harming themselves and those who are threatening to harm themselves and who have the means to do so are at immediate risk
Immediate risk to others	An initial view of the risk of harm to others can be judged by looking at posture (tense, clenched), speech (loud, using threatening words) and motor behaviour (restless, pacing, lunging at others). Immediate risk should be assumed if weapons and potential victims are available and no controls are already in place
Altered conscious level ***not*** wholly attributable to alcohol	A patient who is not fully alert, with a history of alcohol ingestion, and whom there may be other causes of reduced conscious level
Inadequate history	If there is no clear and unequivocal history of acute alcohol ingestion, and if head injury, drug ingestion, underlying medical condition, etc. cannot be definitely excluded, then the history is inadequate
Altered conscious level wholly attributable to alcohol	A patient who is not fully alert, with a clear history of alcohol ingestion, and in whom there is no doubt that all other causes of reduced conscious level have been excluded
History of head injury	A history of a recent physically traumatic event involving the head. Usually this will be reported by the patient but if the patient has been unconscious this history should be sought from a reliable witness

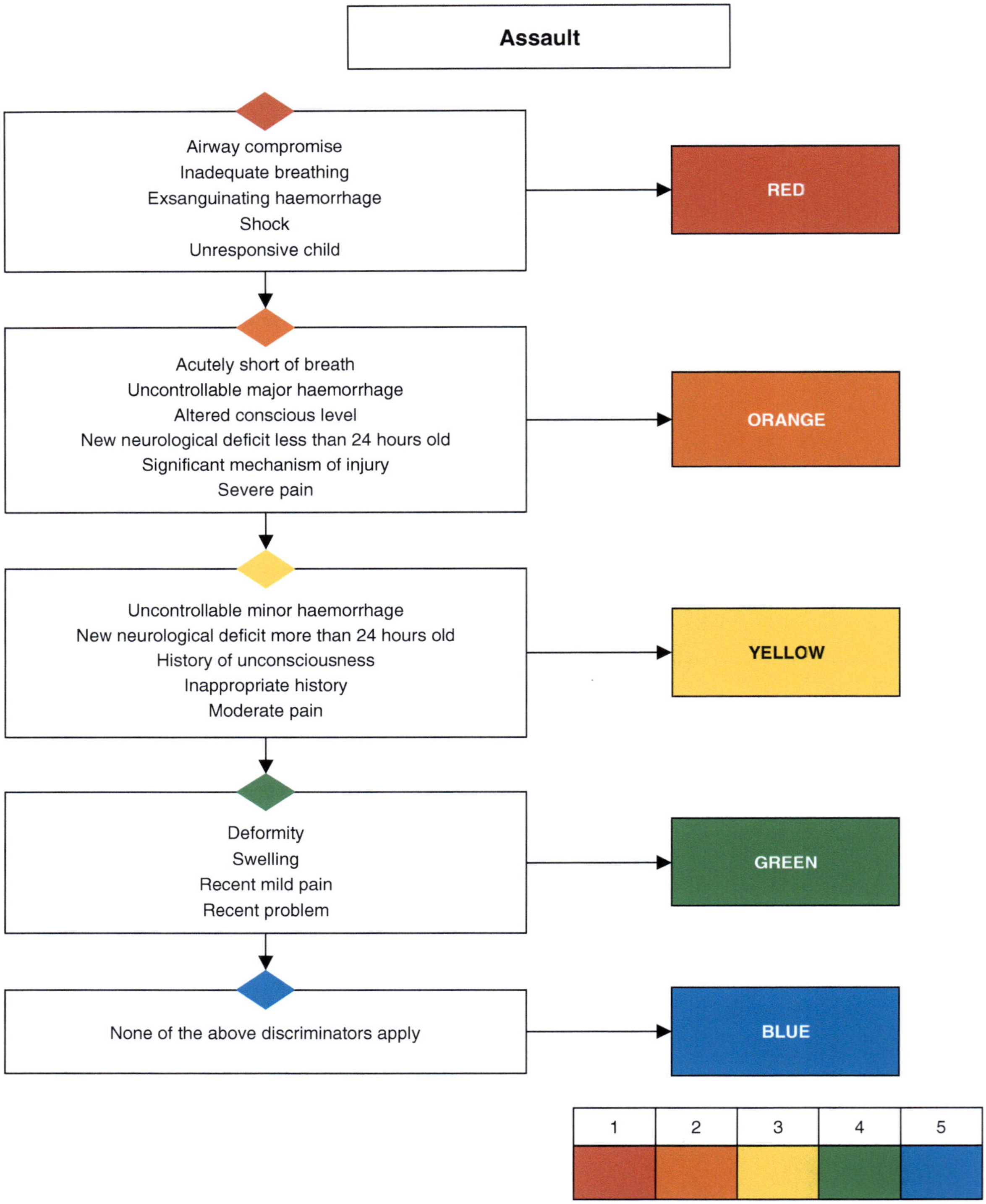
Assault
Airway compromise
Inadequate breathing
Exsanguinating haemorrhage
Shock
Unresponsive child
RED
Acutely short of breath
Uncontrollable major haemorrhage
Altered conscious level
New neurological deficit less than 24 hours old
Significant mechanism of injury
Severe pain
ORANGE
Uncontrollable minor haemorrhage
New neurological deficit more than 24 hours old
History of unconsciousness
Inappropriate history
Moderate pain
YELLOW
Deformity
Swelling
Recent mild pain
Recent problem
GREEN
None of the above discriminators apply
BLUE
1
2
3
4
5

Notes accompanying Assault

Related charts	Chart notes
Head injury Torso injury Wounds	Assault is a common presentation, and patients with non-specific conditions following assault may be triaged using this chart. Patients who have specific injuries are better triaged using the charts that pertain to those injuries. A number of general discriminators are used including *Life threat*, *Haemorrhage* and *Pain*. Specific discriminators are included to identify patients who have a significant history of injury which may indicate a more urgent requirement for treatment

Relevant discriminators	Definition
Acutely short of breath	Shortness of breath that comes on suddenly, or a sudden exacerbation of chronic shortness of breath
New neurological deficit less than 24 hours old	Any loss of neurological function that has come on within the previous 24 hours. This might include altered or lost sensation, weakness of the limbs (either transiently or permanently) and alterations in bladder or bowel function
Significant mechanism of injury	Penetrating injuries (stab or gunshot) and injuries with high energy transfer. In the frail/elderly, low energy transfer such as a fall from standing, may be significant
New neurological deficit more than 24 hours old	Any loss of neurological function including altered or lost sensation, weakness of the limbs (either transiently or permanently) and alterations in bladder or bowel function
Inappropriate history	When the history (story) given does not explain the physical findings it is termed inappropriate. This is important as it is a marker of safeguarding concerns in both adults and children
Deformity	This will always be subjective. Abnormal angulation or rotation is implied
Swelling	An abnormal increase in size

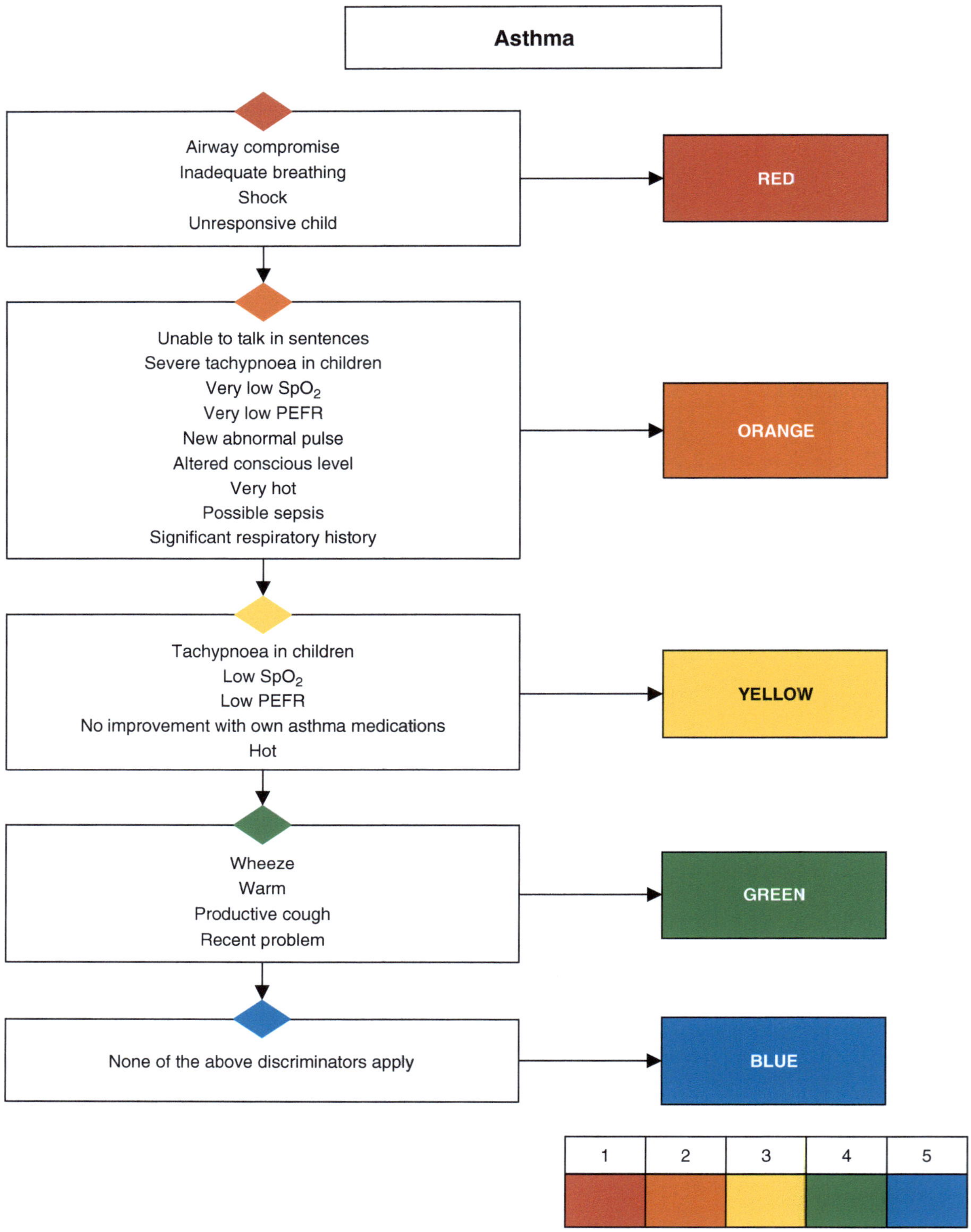
Asthma
Airway compromise
Inadequate breathing
Shock
Unresponsive child
RED
Unable to talk in sentences
Severe tachypnoea in children
Very low SpO_2
Very low PEFR
New abnormal pulse
Altered conscious level
Very hot
Possible sepsis
Significant respiratory history
ORANGE
Tachypnoea in children
Low SpO_2
Low PEFR
No improvement with own asthma medications
Hot
YELLOW
Wheeze
Warm
Productive cough
Recent problem
GREEN
None of the above discriminators apply
BLUE
1
2
3
4
5

Notes accompanying Asthma

Related charts	Chart notes
Allergy Shortness of breath in adults Shortness of breath in children	This chart is intended for use in patients who present with the symptoms and signs of known asthma. The severity of asthmatic patients at presentation varies from those whose lives are threatened to those requiring a repeat prescription of inhalers. A number of general discriminators are used including *Life threat*, *Conscious level (in adults and children)* and *Oxygen saturation*. Specific discriminators are included to indicate those signs and symptoms that indicate severe and life-threatening asthma

Relevant discriminators	Definition
Unable to talk in sentences	Patients who are so breathless that they cannot complete relatively short sentences in one breath
Severe tachypnoea in children	A child less than 1 year with a respiratory rate of 55 breaths per minute or above ***OR*** a child 1 year or above with a respiratory rate of 45 breaths per minute or above
Very low SpO_2	This is a saturation of less than 95% on O_2 therapy or less than 92% on air. The variation in risk according to skin colour necessitates the integration of pulse oximetry with other clinical and patient-reported data
Very low PEFR	The PEFR predicted after consideration of the age and sex of the patient. Some patients may know their 'best' PEFR and this may be used. If the ratio of measured to predicted is less than 33% then this criterion is fulfilled
Significant respiratory history	A history of previous life-threatening episodes of a respiratory condition (e.g. COPD) is significant, as is brittle asthma
Tachypnoea in children	A child less than 1 year with a respiratory rate of 45 breaths per minute or above ***OR*** a child 1 year or above with a respiratory rate of 35 breaths per minute or above
Low SpO_2	This is a saturation of less than 95% on air. The variation in risk according to skin colour necessitates the integration of pulse oximetry with other clinical and patient-reported data
Low PEFR	The PEFR predicted after consideration of the age and sex of the patient. Some patients may know their 'best' PEFR and this may be used. If the ratio of measured to predicted is less than 50% then this criterion is fulfilled
No improvement with own asthma medications	This history should be available from the patient. A failure to improve with bronchodilator therapy given by the GP or paramedic is equally significant
Wheeze	This can be audible wheeze or a feeling of wheeze. Very severe airway obstruction is silent (no air can move)
Productive cough	A cough that is productive of phlegm, whatever the colour

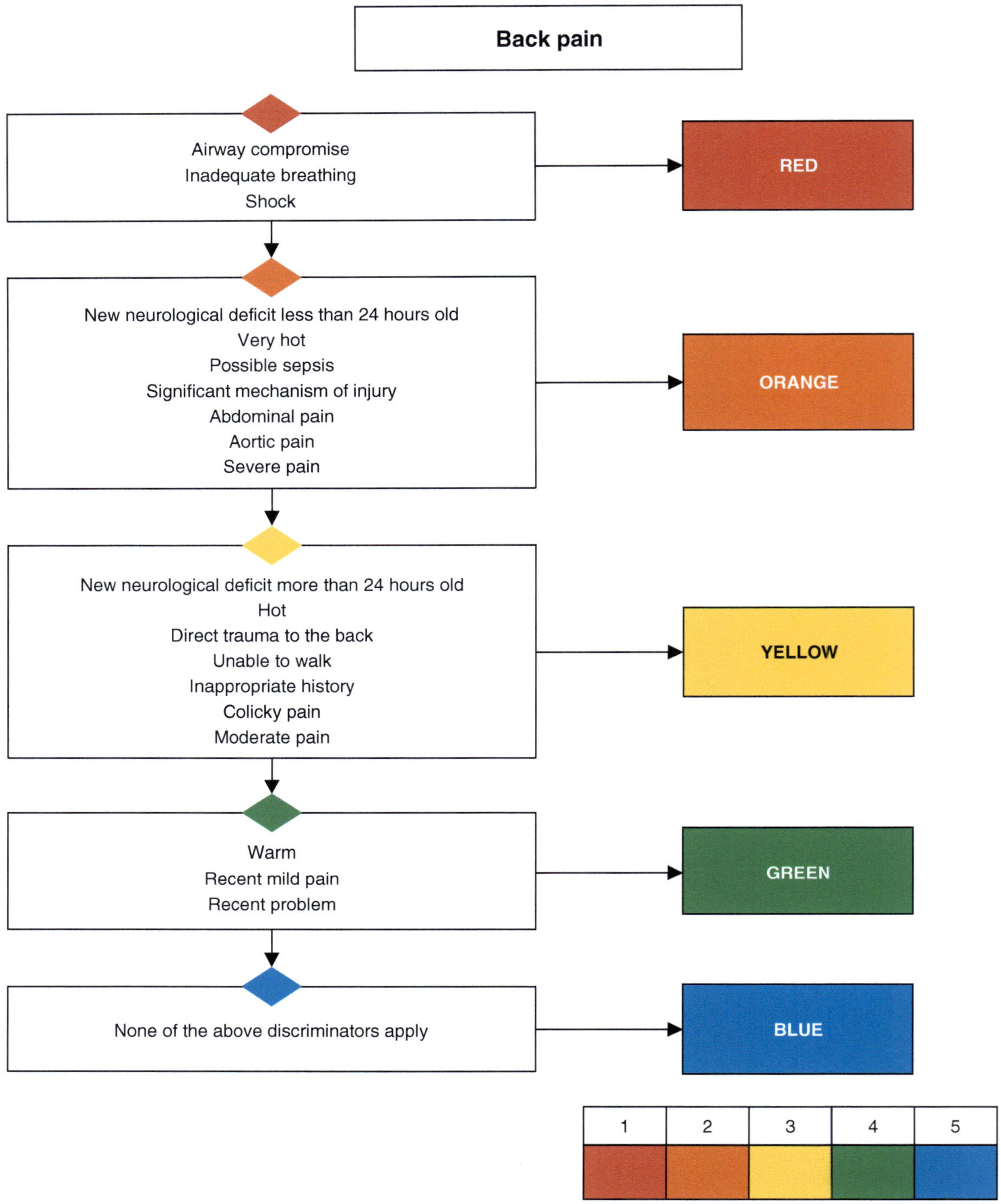
Back pain
Airway compromise
Inadequate breathing
Shock
RED
New neurological deficit less than 24 hours old
Very hot
Possible sepsis
Significant mechanism of injury
Abdominal pain
Aortic pain
Severe pain
ORANGE
New neurological deficit more than 24 hours old
Hot
Direct trauma to the back
Unable to walk
Inappropriate history
Colicky pain
Moderate pain
YELLOW
Warm
Recent mild pain
Recent problem
GREEN
None of the above discriminators apply
BLUE
1
2
3
4
5

Notes accompanying Back pain

Related charts	Chart notes
Abdominal pain in adults Abdominal pain in children Neck pain	Back pain may present to urgent and emergency care either as an acute event or as an acute exacerbation of a chronic problem. A number of general discriminators are used including *Life threat*, *Pain* and *Temperature*. Specific discriminators have been selected in order to allow for appropriate categorisation of more urgent problems. In particular, discriminators are included to allow appropriate classification of abdominal aneurysm and patients with neurological signs and symptoms following disc prolapse

Relevant discriminators	Definition
New neurological deficit less than 24 hours old	Any loss of neurological function that has come on within the previous 24 hours. This might include altered or lost sensation, weakness of the limbs (either transiently or permanently) and alterations in bladder or bowel function
Significant mechanism of injury	Penetrating injuries (stab or gunshot) and injuries with high energy transfer. In the frail/elderly, low energy transfer such as a fall from standing may be significant
Abdominal pain	Any pain felt in the abdomen. Abdominal pain associated with back pain may indicate abdominal aortic aneurysm, while association with PV bleeding may indicate ectopic pregnancy or miscarriage
Aortic pain	The onset of symptoms is sudden and the leading symptom is severe abdominal or chest pain. The pain may be described as sharp, stabbing or ripping in character. Classically aortic chest pain is felt around the sternum and then radiates to the shoulder blades, aortic abdominal pain is felt in the centre of the abdomen and radiates to the back. The pain may get better or even vanish and then recur elsewhere. Over time, pain may also be felt in the arms, neck, lower jaw, stomach or hips
New neurological deficit more than 24 hours old	Any loss of neurological function including altered or lost sensation, weakness of the limbs (either transiently or permanently) and alterations in bladder or bowel function
Direct trauma to the back	This may be top to bottom (loading), for instance when people fall and land on their feet, bending (forwards, backwards or to the side) or twisting
Unable to walk	It is important to try and distinguish between patients who have pain and difficulty walking and those who cannot walk. Only the latter can be said to be unable to walk
Colicky pain	Pain that comes and goes in waves. Renal colic tends to come and go over 20 minutes or so

Behaving strangely

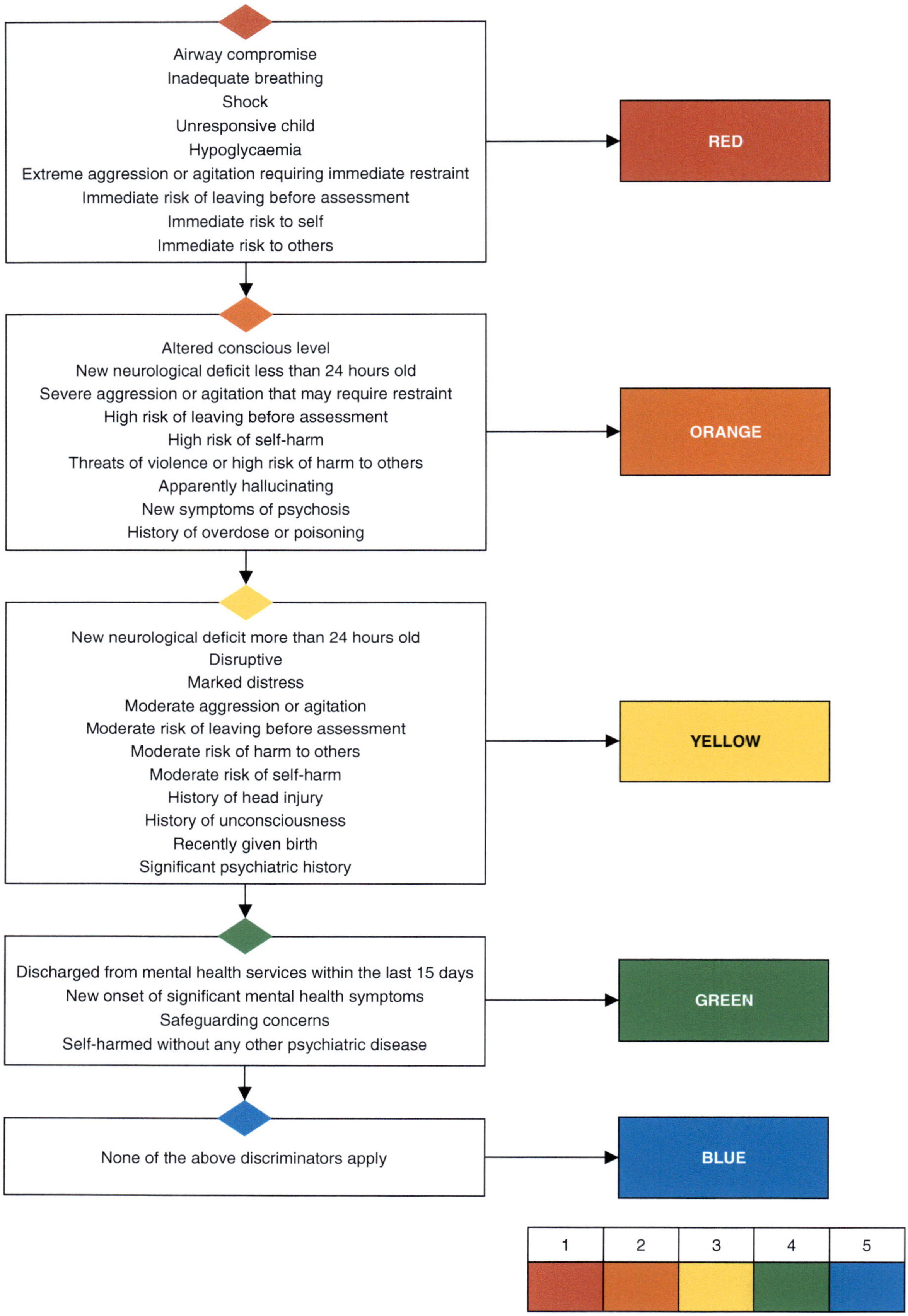

Notes accompanying Behaving strangely

Related charts	Chart notes
Apparently drunk Mental illness	Patients who are behaving strangely may have either a psychiatric or a physical cause for their presentation. This chart is designed to allow the accurate prioritisation of both of these groups of patients. A number of general discriminators have been used, including *Life threat* and *Conscious level*. Specific discriminators are used and in particular the concepts of risk of harm to others and risks of self-harm are introduced

Relevant discriminators	Definition
Hypoglycaemia	Glucose less than 3 mmol/l
Extreme aggression or agitation requiring immediate restraint	Aggression and agitation of such a degree that immediate restraint is required to manage the risk of harm to self or others
Immediate risk of leaving before assessment	Active, credible attempts to leave prior to assessment pose an immediate risk
Immediate risk to self	An initial view of the risk of harm to self can be formed by considering the patient's behaviour. Patients who are actively harming themselves and those who are threatening to harm themselves and who have the means to do so are at immediate risk
Immediate risk to others	An initial view of the risk of harm to others can be judged by looking at posture (tense, clenched), speech (loud, using threatening words) and motor behaviour (restless, pacing, lunging at others). Immediate risk should be assumed if weapons and potential victims are available and no controls are already in place
Apparently hallucinating	Patients who are apparently hallucinating may appear distracted and may appear to react to stimuli (primarily visual and auditory) that are not apparent to anyone else
New symptoms of psychosis	Active new symptoms of psychosis with no insight such as hallucinations, delusions and/or paranoia
History of overdose or poisoning	This information may come from others or may be deduced if medication is missing
Recently given birth	A patient who has given birth within the past 3 months
Significant psychiatric history	A history of a major psychiatric illness or event
Discharged from mental health services within the last 15 days	Any patient who has been discharged from an active period of care under mental health services (in hospital or in the community) within the last 15 days
New onset of significant mental health symptoms	Any new mental health symptoms not already taken into account

Bites and stings

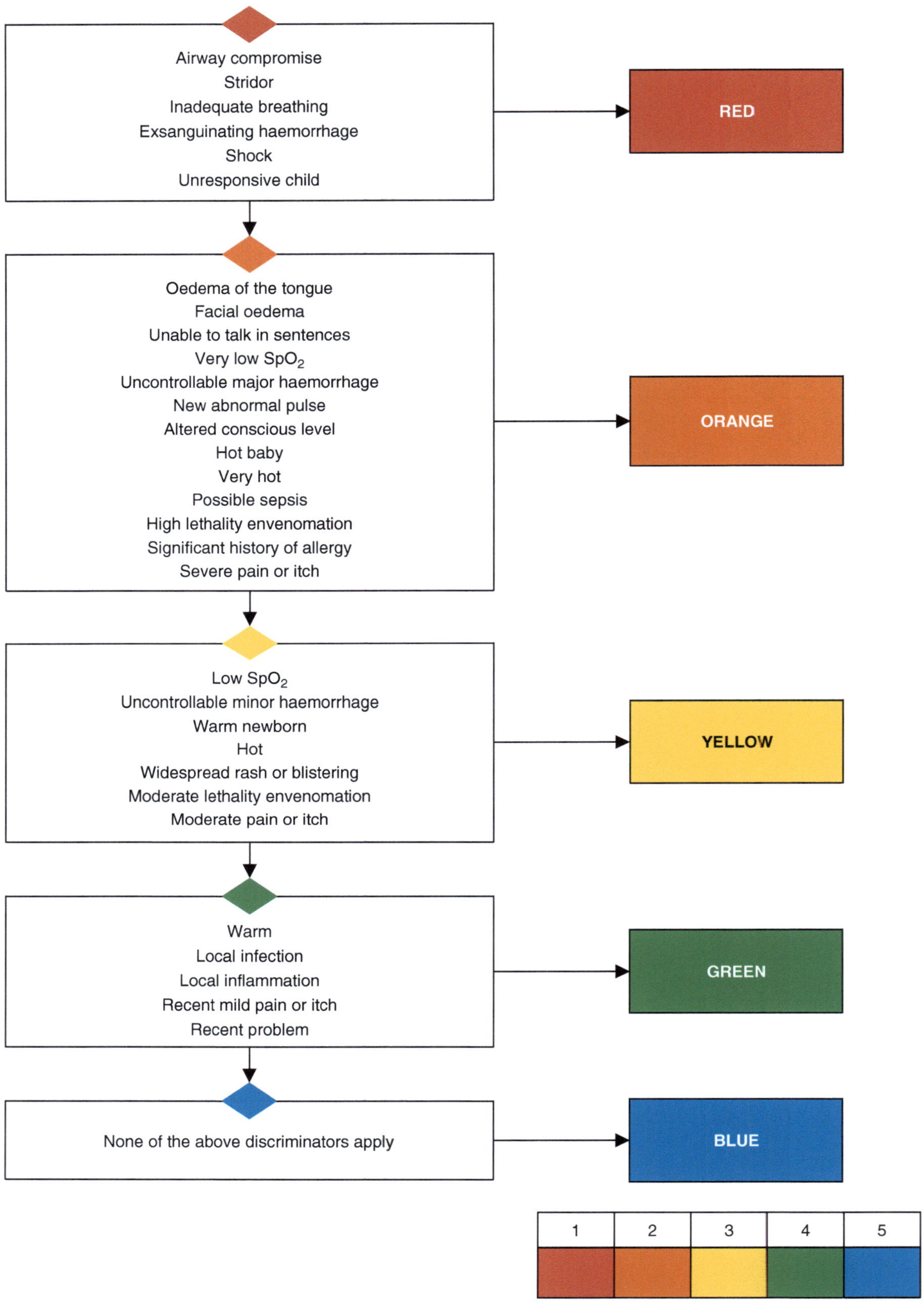

Notes accompanying Bites and stings

Related charts	Chart notes
Abscesses and local infections Allergy	This chart is designed to allow accurate prioritisation of patients who present following bites and stings. Bites may, of course, range from those delivered by insects to those delivered by large animals; therefore, there is a complete range of priority covered by this presentation. A number of general discriminators are used including *Life threat*, *Haemorrhage* and *Pain*. Specific discriminators have been added to the chart to allow accurate identification of patients requiring more urgent treatment because of more severe injury or the development of allergic reactions

Relevant discriminators	Definition
Stridor	This may be an inspiratory or expiratory noise, or both. Stridor is heard best on breathing with the mouth open
Oedema of the tongue	Swelling of the tongue of any degree
Facial oedema	Diffuse swelling around the face, usually involving the lips
Unable to talk in sentences	Patients who are so breathless that they cannot complete relatively short sentences in one breath
High lethality envenomation	Lethality is the potential of the envenomation to cause harm. Local knowledge may allow identification of the venomous creature, but advice may be required. If in doubt, assume a high risk
Significant history of allergy	A known sensitivity with severe reaction (e.g. to nuts or bee sting) is significant
Widespread rash or blistering	Any rash or blistering eruption covering more than 10% of the body surface area
Local infection	Local infection usually manifests as inflammation (pain, swelling and redness) confined to a particular site or area, with or without a collection of pus
Local inflammation	Local inflammation will involve pain, swelling and redness confined to a particular site or area

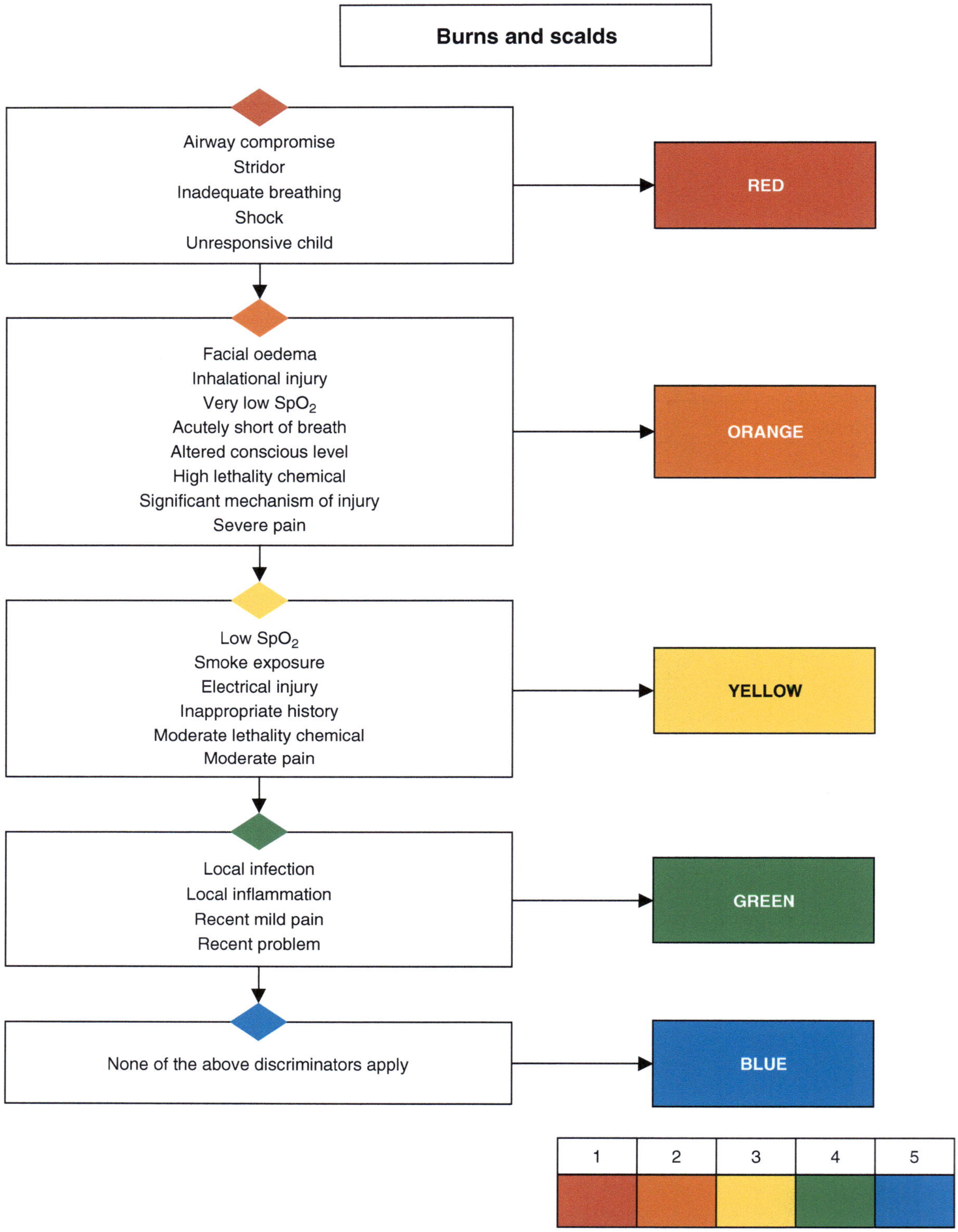
Burns and scalds
Airway compromise
Stridor
Inadequate breathing
Shock
Unresponsive child
RED
Facial oedema
Inhalational injury
Very low SpO_2
Acutely short of breath
Altered conscious level
High lethality chemical
Significant mechanism of injury
Severe pain
ORANGE
Low SpO_2
Smoke exposure
Electrical injury
Inappropriate history
Moderate lethality chemical
Moderate pain
YELLOW
Local infection
Local inflammation
Recent mild pain
Recent problem
GREEN
None of the above discriminators apply
BLUE
1
2
3
4
5

Notes accompanying Burns and scalds

Related charts	Chart notes
None	There is a complete range of severity with this presentation and the chart is designed to allow accurate identification of patients within each category. A number of general discriminators are used including *Life threat*, *Conscious level* and *Pain*. Specific discriminators have been added to allow identification of patients who have suffered inhalation injury, and those in whom the mechanism suggests that further investigation and treatment may be appropriate

Relevant discriminators	Definition
Stridor	This may be an inspiratory or expiratory noise, or both. Stridor is heard best on breathing with the mouth open
Facial oedema	Diffuse swelling around the face, usually involving the lips
Inhalational injury	A history of being confined in a smoke-filled space is the most reliable indicator of smoke inhalation. Carbon deposits around the mouth and nose and hoarse voice may be present. History is also the most reliable way of diagnosing inhalation of chemicals – there will not necessarily be any signs
High lethality chemical	Lethality is the potential of the chemical to cause harm. Advice may be required to establish the level of risk. If in doubt, assume a high risk
Smoke exposure	Smoke inhalation should be assumed if the patient has been confined in a smoke-filled space. Physical signs such as oral or nasal soot are less reliable but significant if present
Electrical injury	Any injury caused or possibly caused by an electric current. This includes AC and DC and both artificial and natural sources
Moderate lethality chemical	Lethality is the potential of the chemical to cause harm. Advice may be required to establish the level of risk. If in doubt, assume a high risk
Local infection	Local infection usually manifests as inflammation (pain, swelling and redness) confined to a particular site or area, with or without a collection of pus

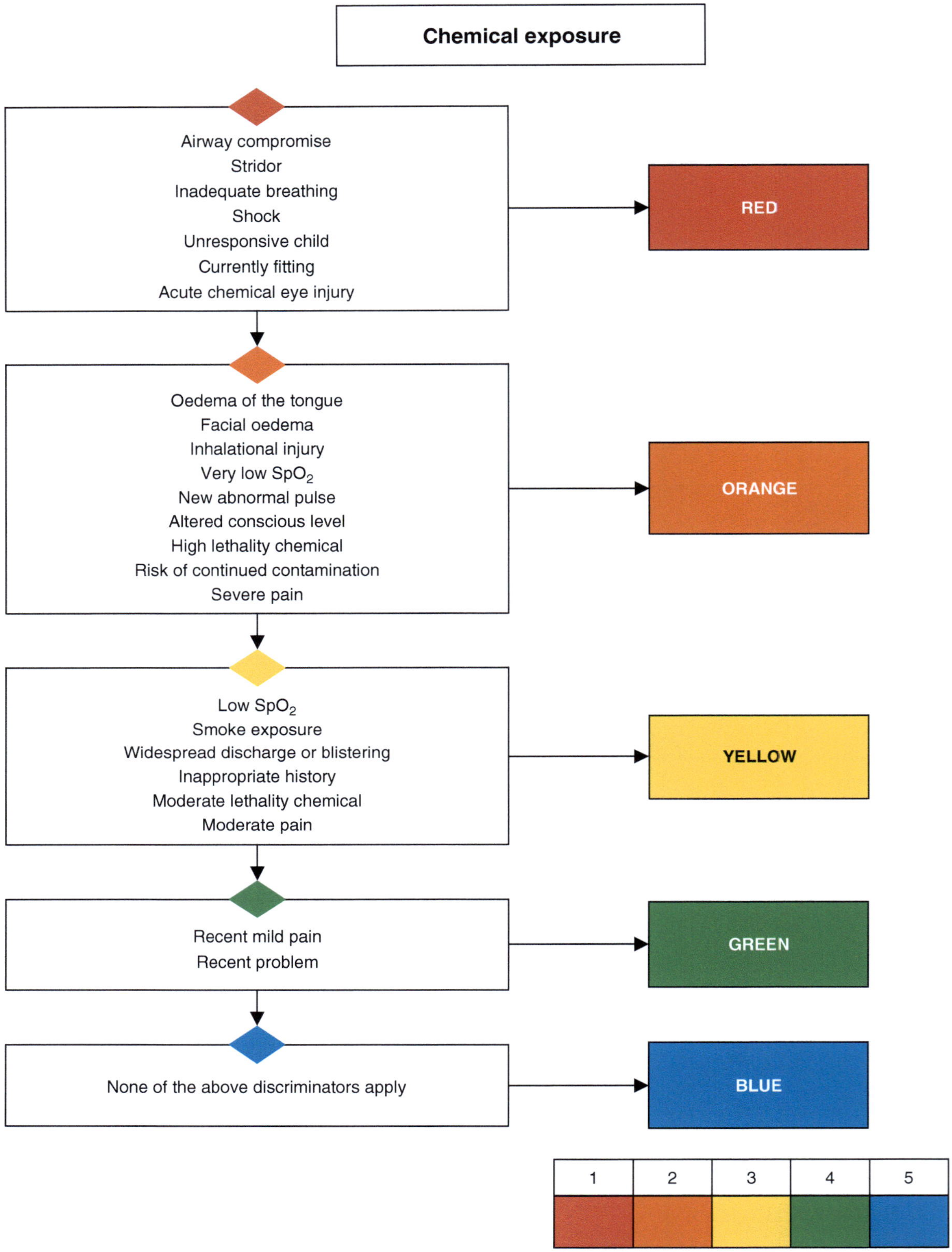
Chemical exposure
Airway compromise
Stridor
Inadequate breathing
Shock
Unresponsive child
Currently fitting
Acute chemical eye injury
RED
Oedema of the tongue
Facial oedema
Inhalational injury
Very low SpO_2
New abnormal pulse
Altered conscious level
High lethality chemical
Risk of continued contamination
Severe pain
ORANGE
Low SpO_2
Smoke exposure
Widespread discharge or blistering
Inappropriate history
Moderate lethality chemical
Moderate pain
YELLOW
Recent mild pain
Recent problem
GREEN
None of the above discriminators apply
BLUE
1
2
3
4
5

Notes accompanying Chemical exposure

Related charts	Chart notes
Shortness of breath in adults Shortness of breath in children	While this presentation is not common, it is important because it is often the chief complaint of the patient. The signs and symptoms do not necessarily fit easily into any other presentational group. A number of general discriminators are used including *Life threat*, *Conscious level*, *Pain* and *Oxygen saturation*. Specific discriminators, which include those for the shortness of breath, have been added to appropriate categories. *Acute chemical eye injury* appears in the RED category and *Risk of continued contamination* appears in the ORANGE

Relevant discriminators	Definition
Stridor	This may be an inspiratory or expiratory noise, or both. Stridor is heard best on breathing with the mouth open
Acute chemical eye injury	Any substance splashed into or placed into the eye within the past 12 hours that caused stinging, burning or reduced vision should be assumed to have caused chemical injury
Oedema of the tongue	Swelling of the tongue of any degree
Facial oedema	Diffuse swelling around the face, usually involving the lips
Inhalational injury	A history of being confined in a smoke-filled space is the most reliable indicator of smoke inhalation. Carbon deposits around the mouth and nose and hoarse voice may be present. History is also the most reliable way of diagnosing inhalation of chemicals – there will not necessarily be any signs
High lethality chemical	Lethality is the potential of the chemical to cause harm. Advice may be required to establish the level of risk. If in doubt, assume a high risk
Risk of continued contamination	If chemical exposure is likely to continue (usually due to lack of adequate decontamination) then this discriminator applies. Risks to healthcare workers must not be forgotten if this situation occurs
Smoke exposure	Smoke inhalation should be assumed if the patient has been confined in a smoke-filled space. Physical signs such as oral or nasal soot are less reliable but significant if present
Widespread discharge or blistering	Any discharging or blistering eruption covering more than 10% of the body surface area.
Moderate lethality chemical	Lethality is the potential of the chemical to cause harm. Advice may be required to establish the level of risk. If in doubt, assume a high risk

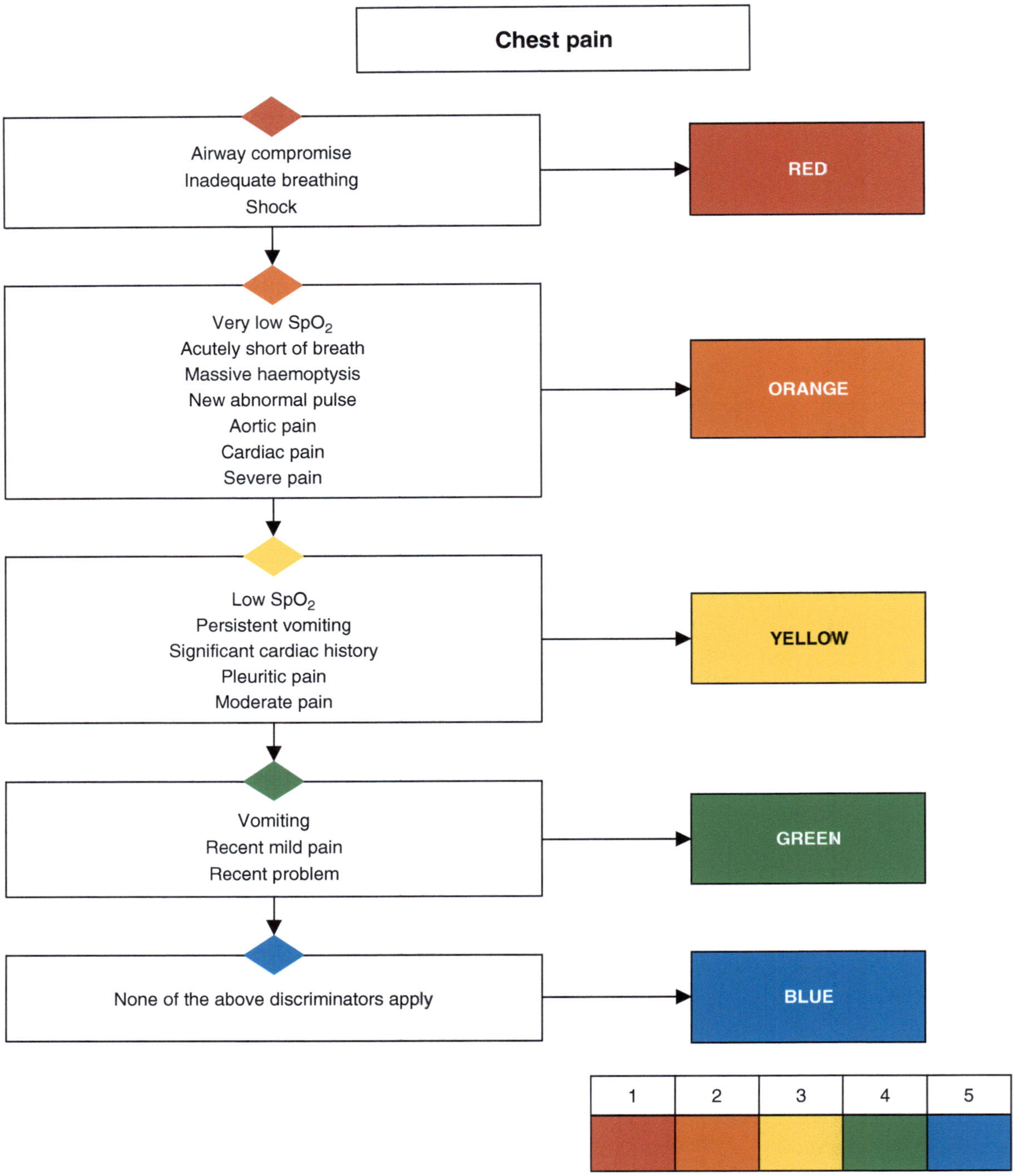
Chest pain
Airway compromise
Inadequate breathing
Shock
RED
Very low SpO_2
Acutely short of breath
Massive haemoptysis
New abnormal pulse
Aortic pain
Cardiac pain
Severe pain
ORANGE
Low SpO_2
Persistent vomiting
Significant cardiac history
Pleuritic pain
Moderate pain
YELLOW
Vomiting
Recent mild pain
Recent problem
GREEN
None of the above discriminators apply
BLUE
1
2
3
4
5

Notes accompanying Chest pain

Related charts	Chart notes
None	Chest pain is a common presentation to urgent and emergency care departments, forming some 2–5% of all patient contacts. Causes of chest pain may vary from acute myocardial infarction to muscular irritation, and appropriate categorisation is paramount. A number of general discriminators are used including *Life threat* and *Pain*. Specific discriminators include the nature and severity of pain (cardiac or pleuritic) and abnormalities of pulse

Relevant discriminators	Definition
Acutely short of breath	Shortness of breath that comes on suddenly, or a sudden exacerbation of chronic shortness of breath
Massive haemoptysis	Coughing up large amounts of fresh or clotted blood. Not to be confused with streaks of blood in saliva
New abnormal pulse	A bradycardia (less than 60/min in adults), a tachycardia (more than 100/min in adults) or an irregular rhythm. Age-appropriate definitions of bradycardia and tachycardia should be used in children
Aortic pain	The onset of symptoms is sudden and the leading symptom is severe abdominal or chest pain. The pain may be described as sharp, stabbing or ripping in character. Classically, aortic chest pain is felt around the sternum and then radiates to the shoulder blades; aortic abdominal pain is felt in the centre of the abdomen and radiates to the back. The pain may get better or even vanish and then recur elsewhere. Over time, pain may also be felt in the arms, neck, lower jaw, stomach or hips
Cardiac pain	Classically, a severe dull 'gripping' or 'heavy' pain in the centre of the chest, radiating to the left arm or to the neck. Maybe associated with sweating and nausea. Some patients may be less likely to seek medical attention and treatment quickly, despite the warning signs
Persistent vomiting	Vomiting that is continuous or that occurs without any respite between episodes
Significant cardiac history	A known recurrent dysrhythmia that has life-threatening effects is significant, as is a known cardiac condition which may deteriorate rapidly
Pleuritic pain	A sharp, localised pain in the chest that worsens on breathing, coughing or sneezing
Vomiting	Any emesis

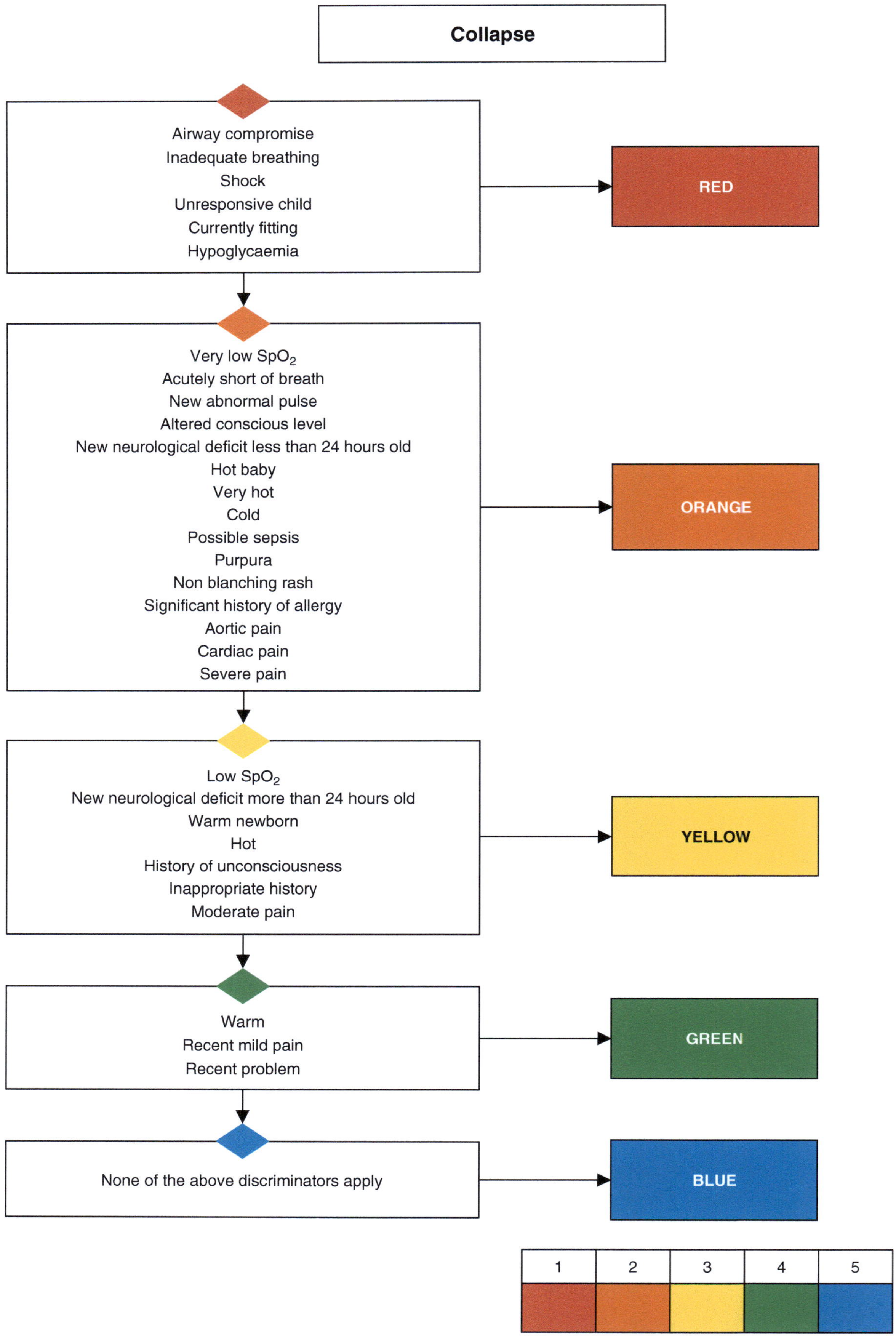
Collapse
Airway compromise
Inadequate breathing
Shock
Unresponsive child
Currently fitting
Hypoglycaemia
RED
Very low SpO_2
Acutely short of breath
New abnormal pulse
Altered conscious level
New neurological deficit less than 24 hours old
Hot baby
Very hot
Cold
Possible sepsis
Purpura
Non blanching rash
Significant history of allergy
Aortic pain
Cardiac pain
Severe pain
ORANGE
Low SpO_2
New neurological deficit more than 24 hours old
Warm newborn
Hot
History of unconsciousness
Inappropriate history
Moderate pain
YELLOW
Warm
Recent mild pain
Recent problem
GREEN
None of the above discriminators apply
BLUE
1
2
3
4
5

Notes accompanying Collapse

Related charts	Chart notes
Apparently drunk Falls Fits Unwell adult Unwell baby up to 12 months Unwell child	Presentation with collapse is not uncommon in an urgent and emergency care department, and this chart is designed to allow rapid triage of patients who present in this way. A number of general discriminators are used including *Life threat*, *Conscious level*, *Pain* and *Temperature*. Specific discriminators have been added to the chart to try and rule out more serious pathology. As with all charts, those pathologies (such as myocardial infarction) which can potentially benefit from early intervention are deliberately categorised highly

Relevant discriminators	Definition
Hypoglycaemia	Glucose less than 3 mmol/l
Very low SpO_2	This is a saturation of less than 95% on O_2 therapy or less than 92% on air. The variation in risk according to skin colour necessitates the integration of pulse oximetry with other clinical and patient-reported data
Acutely short of breath	Shortness of breath that comes on suddenly, or a sudden exacerbation of chronic shortness of breath
New neurological deficit less than 24 hours old	Any loss of neurological function that has come on within the previous 24 hours. This might include altered or lost sensation, weakness of the limbs (either transiently or permanently) and alterations in bladder or bowel function
Possible sepsis	Suspected sepsis in patients who present with altered mental state, low blood pressure (systolic less than 100 mmHg) or raised respiratory rate (rate more than 22 breaths per minute) when using the qSOFA tool for assessment. Other sepsis screening tools may be used instead of qSOFA, and the relevant sepsis markers applied. In children, age-specific physiological tools should be used to determine if possibly septic
Significant history of allergy	A known sensitivity with severe reaction (e.g. to nuts or bee sting) is significant
Aortic pain	The onset of symptoms is sudden and the leading symptom is severe abdominal or chest pain. The pain may be described as sharp, stabbing or ripping in character. Classically, aortic chest pain is felt around the sternum and then radiates to the shoulder blades; aortic abdominal pain is felt in the centre of the abdomen and radiates to the back. The pain may get better or even vanish and then recur elsewhere. Over time, pain may also be felt in the arms, neck, lower jaw, stomach or hips
Cardiac pain	Classically, a severe dull 'gripping' or 'heavy' pain in the centre of the chest, radiating to the left arm or to the neck. Maybe associated with sweating and nausea. Some patients may be less likely to seek medical attention and treatment quickly, despite the warning signs
Low SpO_2	This is a saturation of less than 95% on air. The variation in risk according to skin colour necessitates the integration of pulse oximetry with other clinical and patient-reported data
New neurological deficit more than 24 hours old	Any loss of neurological function including altered or lost sensation, weakness of the limbs (either transiently or permanently) and alterations in bladder or bowel function

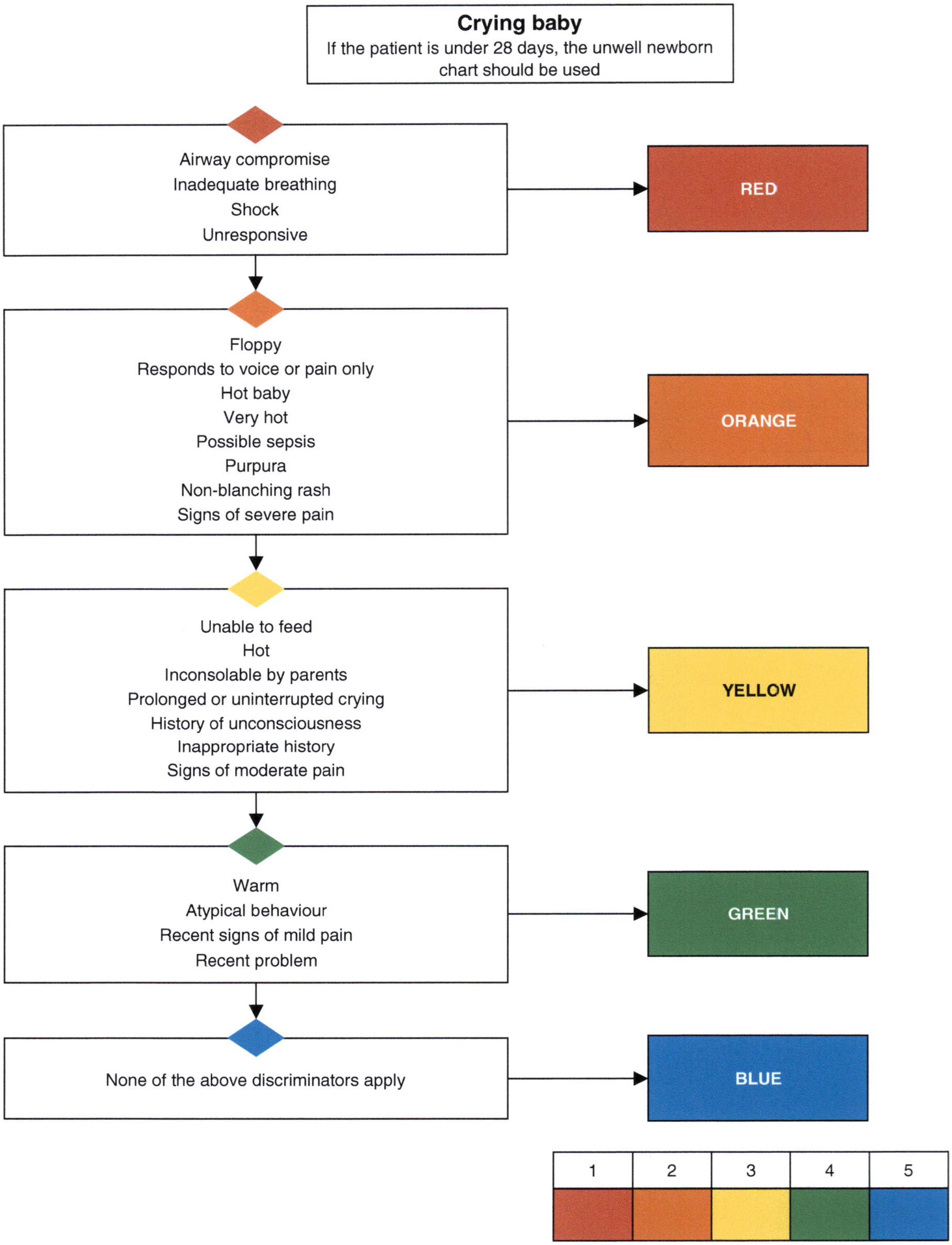
Crying baby
If the patient is under 28 days, the unwell newborn chart should be used
Airway compromise
Inadequate breathing
Shock
Unresponsive
RED
Floppy
Responds to voice or pain only
Hot baby
Very hot
Possible sepsis
Purpura
Non-blanching rash
Signs of severe pain
ORANGE
Unable to feed
Hot
Inconsolable by parents
Prolonged or uninterrupted crying
History of unconsciousness
Inappropriate history
Signs of moderate pain
YELLOW
Warm
Atypical behaviour
Recent signs of mild pain
Recent problem
GREEN
None of the above discriminators apply
BLUE
1
2
3
4
5

Notes accompanying Crying baby

Related charts	**Chart notes**
Irritable child Unwell baby up to 12 months Unwell child Unwell newborn up to 28 days Worried parent	This chart is designed to allow accurate prioritisation of children who are presented by their parents or carer, with a chief complaint of crying. A number of general discriminators have been used including *Life threat*, *Conscious level* and *Pain*. Specific discriminators include those that allow recognition of more specific pathologies such as septicaemia, or that indicate that a more serious pathology might exist. If the patient is under 28 days, the Unwell newborn chart should be used

Relevant discriminators	**Definition**
Floppy	Parents may describe their children as floppy. Tone is generally reduced – the most noticeable sign is often lolling of the head
Responds to voice or pain only	Responds to painful stimuli, which could include standard peripheral stimuli – a pen or pencil is used to apply pressure to the finger or nail bed. The stimulus should not be applied to the toes since a spinal reflex may cause flexion even in brain death. Central stimuli such as trapezius squeeze or supraorbital ridge pressure can be used but clinicians should be aware reflex grimacing may occur It is not necessary to shout the patient's name. Children may fail to respond because they are afraid
Signs of severe pain	Young children and babies in severe pain cannot complain. They will usually cry out continuously and inconsolably and be tachycardic. They may well exhibit signs such as pallor and sweating
Unable to feed	This is usually reported by the parents. Children who will not take any solid or liquid (as appropriate) by mouth
Inconsolable by parents	Children whose crying or distress does not respond to attempts by their parents to comfort them
Prolonged or uninterrupted crying	A child who has cried continuously for 2 hours or more
Atypical behaviour	Children who are behaving in a way that is not usual in the given situation. The carers will often volunteer this information. Such children are often referred to as fractious or 'out of sorts'

Dental problems

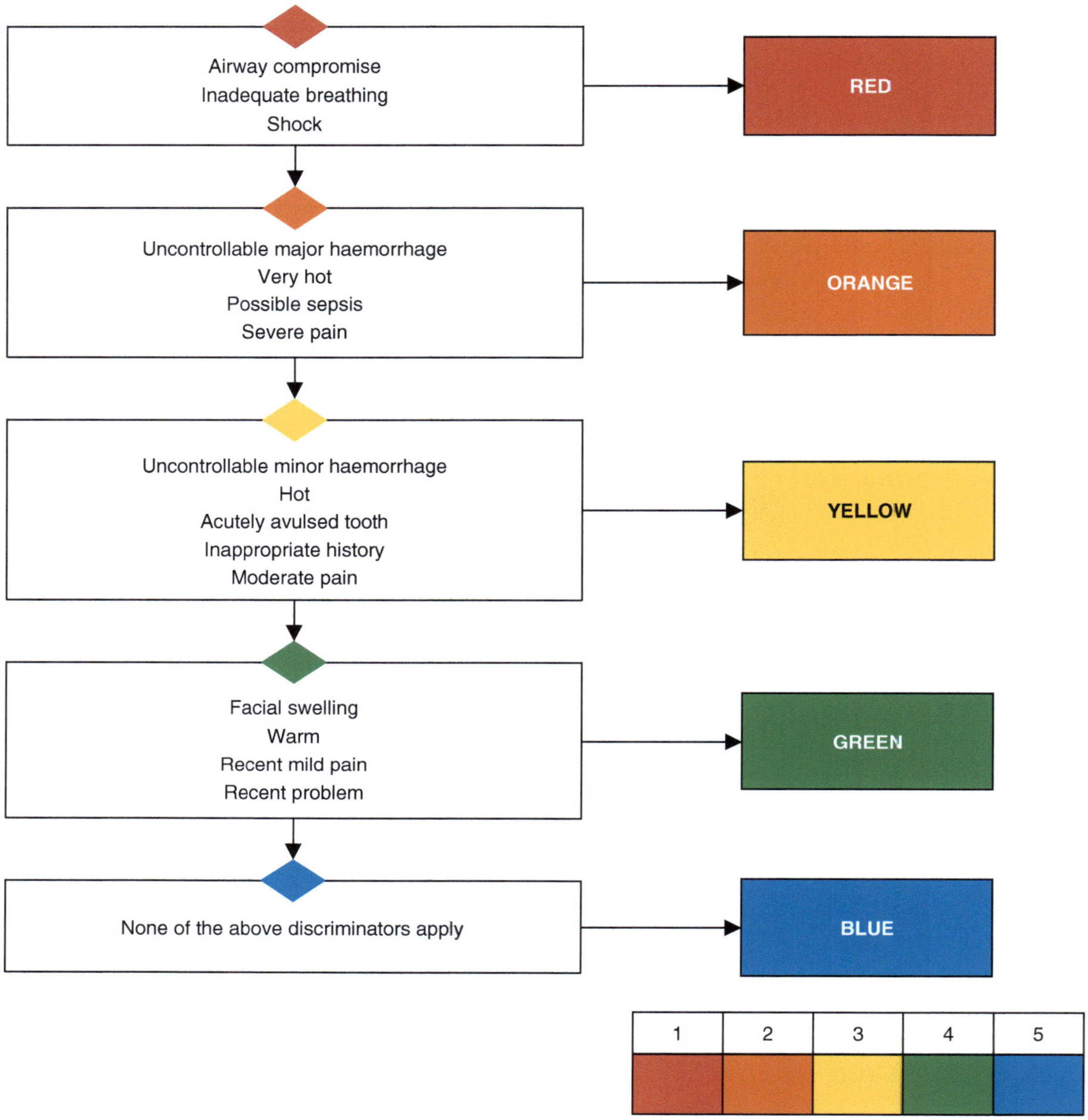

Notes accompanying Dental problems

Related charts	Chart notes
Facial problems	This chart is designed to allow accurate prioritisation of patients presenting problems affecting the teeth or gums. A number of general discriminators have been used including *Life threat*, *Pain*, *Haemorrhage* and *Temperature*. Acute avulsion of a tooth has been included in the urgent (YELLOW) category since speed of reimplantation affects outcome. It is important to ensure that preconceptions about disposal do not affect accurate triage of patients with these presentations

Relevant discriminators	Definition
Possible sepsis	Suspected sepsis in patients who present with altered mental state, low blood pressure (systolic less than 100 mmHg) or raised respiratory rate (rate more than 22 breaths per minute) when using the qSOFA tool for assessment. Other sepsis screening tools may be used instead of qSOFA, and the relevant sepsis markers applied. In children, age-specific physiological tools should be used to determine if possibly septic
Acutely avulsed tooth	A tooth that has been avulsed intact within the previous 24 hours
Facial swelling	Swelling around the face which may be localised or diffuse

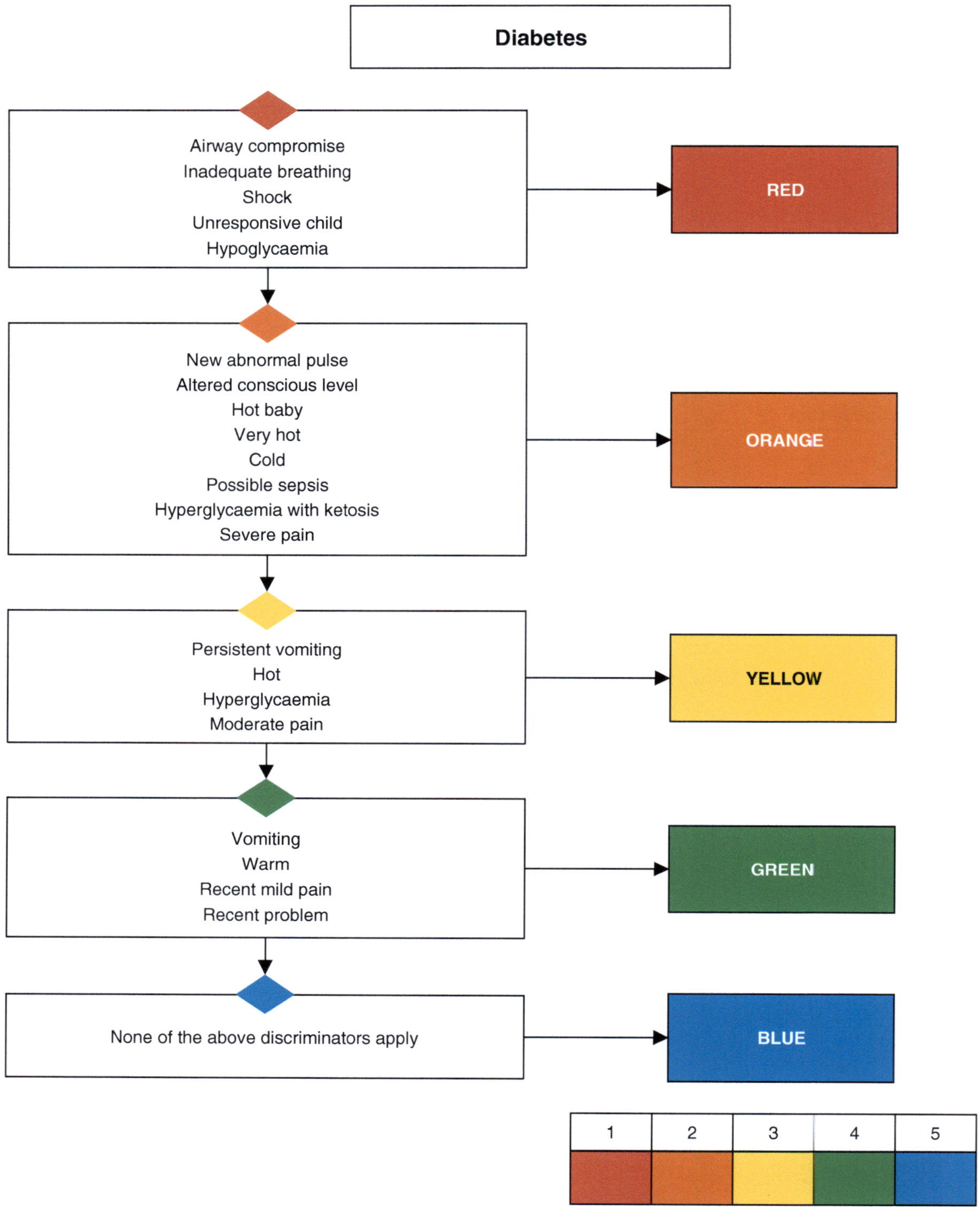
Diabetes
Airway compromise
Inadequate breathing
Shock
Unresponsive child
Hypoglycaemia
RED
New abnormal pulse
Altered conscious level
Hot baby
Very hot
Cold
Possible sepsis
Hyperglycaemia with ketosis
Severe pain
ORANGE
Persistent vomiting
Hot
Hyperglycaemia
Moderate pain
YELLOW
Vomiting
Warm
Recent mild pain
Recent problem
GREEN
None of the above discriminators apply
BLUE
1
2
3
4
5

Notes accompanying Diabetes

Related charts	Chart notes
None	This chart is designed to allow categorisation of patients who present with known cases of diabetes. A number of general discriminators are used including *Life threat*, *Conscious level (both adult and child)*, *Blood glucose level* and *Temperature*

Relevant discriminators	Definition
Hypoglycaemia	Glucose less than 3 mmol/l
Possible sepsis	Suspected sepsis in patients who present with altered mental state, low blood pressure (systolic less than 100 mmHg) or raised respiratory rate (rate more than 22 breaths per minute) when using the qSOFA tool for assessment. Other sepsis screening tools may be used instead of qSOFA, and the relevant sepsis markers applied. In children, age-specific physiological tools should be used to determine if possibly septic
Hyperglycaemia with ketosis	Glucose greater than 11 mmol/l with urinary ketones or signs of acidosis (deep sighing respiration, etc.) Glucose greater than 11 mmol with the presence of ketones. If unable to check for ketones, look for clinical signs of acidosis which may include deep rapid breathing, vomiting and confusion
Persistent vomiting	Vomiting that is continuous or that occurs without any respite between episodes
Hyperglycaemia	Glucose greater than 17 mmol/l
Vomiting	Any emesis

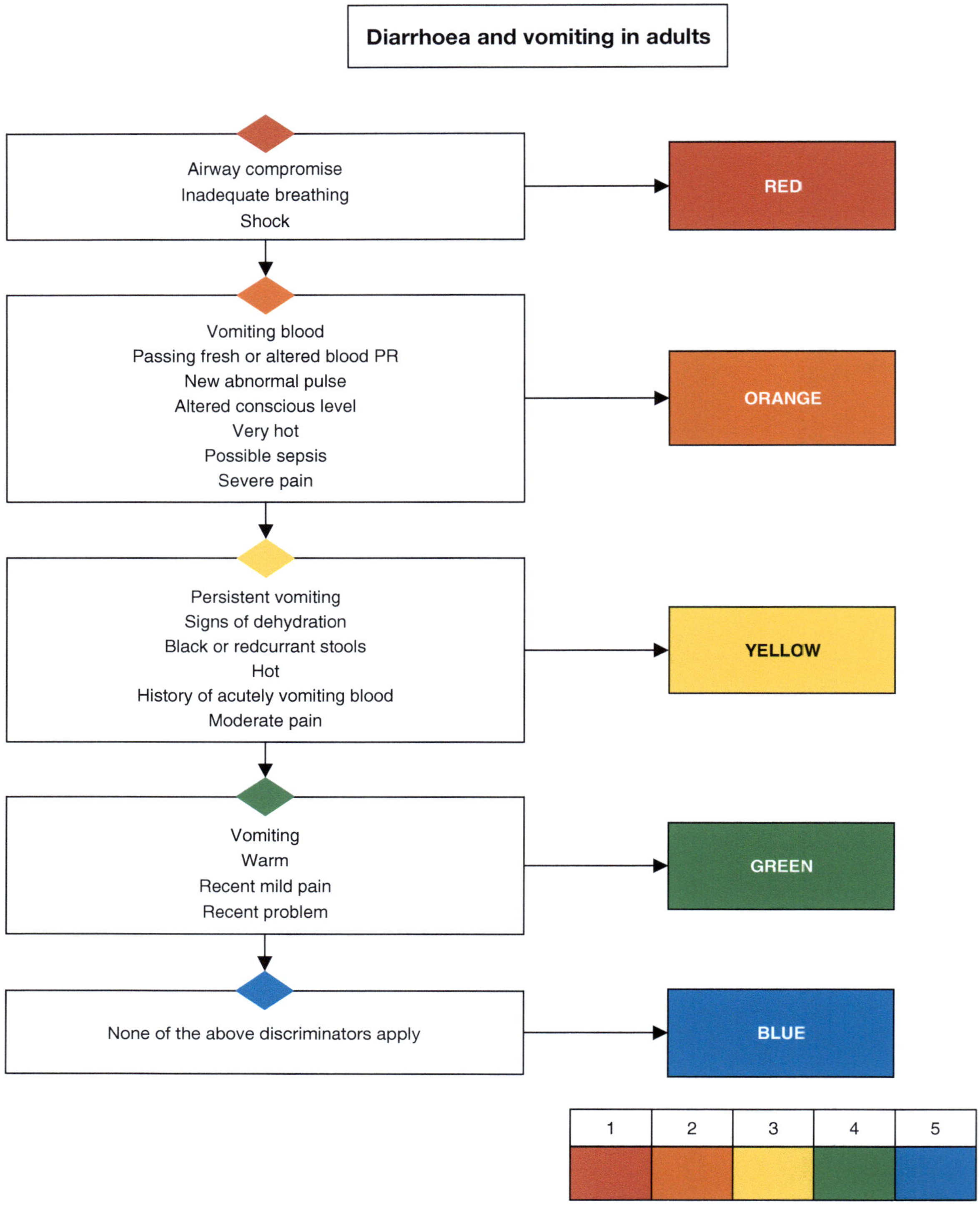
Diarrhoea and vomiting in adults
Airway compromise
Inadequate breathing
Shock
RED
Vomiting blood
Passing fresh or altered blood PR
New abnormal pulse
Altered conscious level
Very hot
Possible sepsis
Severe pain
ORANGE
Persistent vomiting
Signs of dehydration
Black or redcurrant stools
Hot
History of acutely vomiting blood
Moderate pain
YELLOW
Vomiting
Warm
Recent mild pain
Recent problem
GREEN
None of the above discriminators apply
BLUE
1
2
3
4
5

Notes accompanying Diarrhoea and vomiting in adults

Related charts	Chart notes
Abdominal pain in adults GI bleeding	This chart is designed to allow categorisation of patients who present with diarrhoea and/or vomiting. Most patients who present with diarrhoea or vomiting do not have high priority. However, a number may have serious underlying pathology. A number of general discriminators are used including *Life threat* and *Pain*. Specific discriminators have been included to ensure that patients suffering from GI bleeding, and those with dehydration and other severe effects of diarrhoea and vomiting, are included in the appropriate categories

Relevant discriminators	Definition
Vomiting blood	Vomited blood may be fresh (bright or dark red) or coffee ground in appearance
Passing fresh or altered blood PR	In active massive GI bleeding, dark red blood will be passed PR. As GI transit time increases this becomes darker, eventually becoming melaena
Possible sepsis	Suspected sepsis in patients who present with altered mental state, low blood pressure (systolic less than 100 mmHg) or raised respiratory rate (rate more than 22 breaths per minute) when using the qSOFA tool for assessment. Other sepsis screening tools may be used instead of qSOFA, and the relevant sepsis markers applied. In children, age-specific physiological tools should be used to determine if possibly septic
Persistent vomiting	Vomiting that is continuous or that occurs without any respite between episodes
Signs of dehydration	These include dry tongue, sunken eyes, decreased skin turgor and, in small babies, a sunken anterior fontanelle. Usually associated with a low urine output
Black or redcurrant stools	Any blackness fulfils the criteria of black stool while a dark red stool, classically seen in intussusceptions, is redcurrant stool
History of acutely vomiting blood	Frank haematemesis, vomiting of altered blood (coffee ground) or of blood mixed in the vomit within the past 24 hours
Vomiting	Any emesis

Diarrhoea and vomiting in children

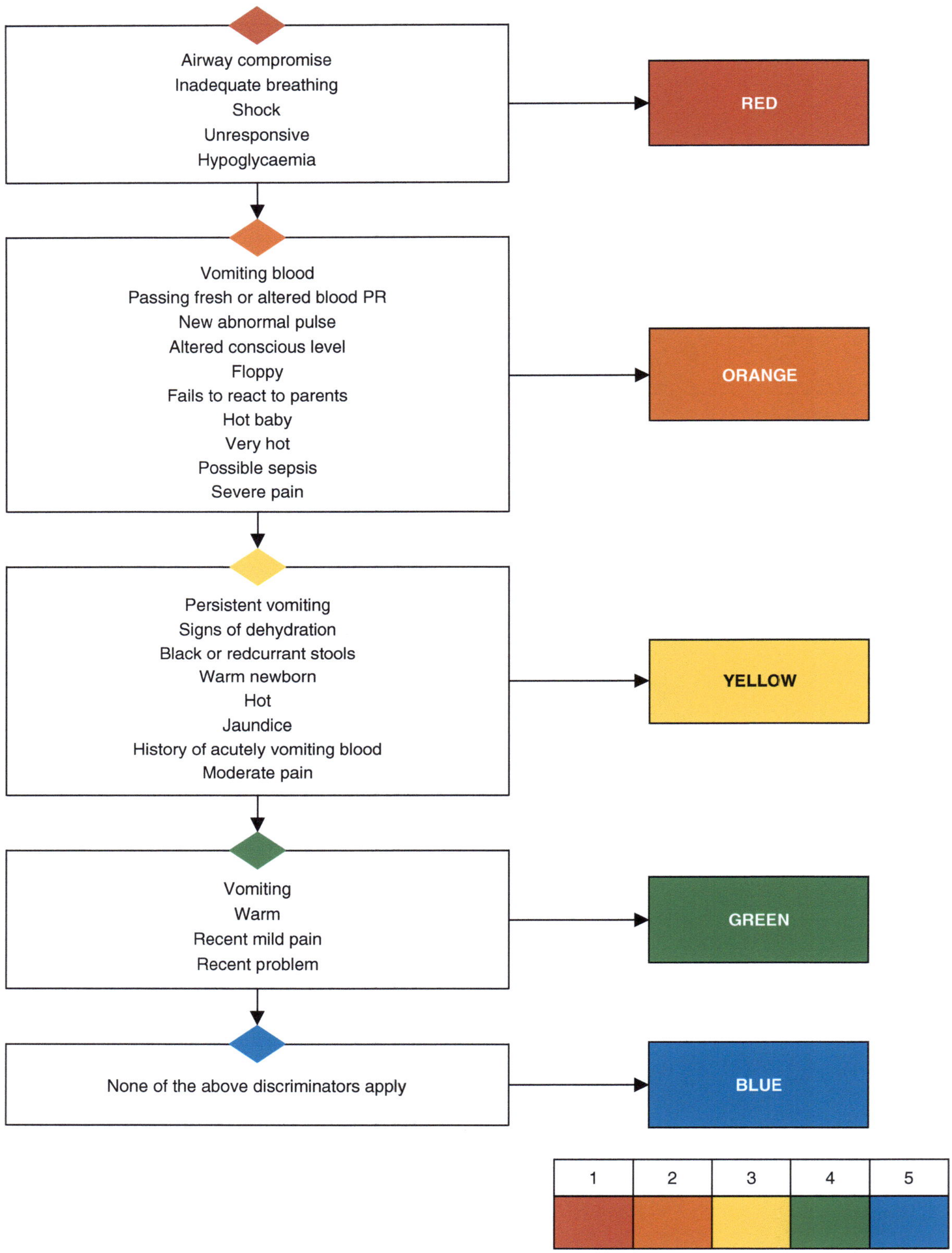

Notes accompanying Diarrhoea and vomiting in children

Related charts	Chart notes
Abdominal pain in children GI bleeding	This chart is designed to allow categorisation of patients who present with diarrhoea and/or vomiting. Most patients who present with diarrhoea or vomiting do not have high priority. However, a number may have serious underlying pathology. A number of general discriminators are used including *Life threat* and *Pain*. Specific discriminators have been included to ensure that patients suffering from GI bleeding, and those with dehydration and other severe effects of diarrhoea and vomiting, are included in the appropriate categories

Relevant discriminators	Definition
Hypoglycaemia	Glucose less than 3 mmol/l
Vomiting blood	Vomited blood may be fresh (bright or dark red) or coffee ground in appearance
Passing fresh or altered blood PR	In active massive GI bleeding, dark red blood will be passed PR. As GI transit time increases this becomes darker, eventually becoming melaena
Floppy	Parents may describe their children as floppy. Tone is generally reduced – the most noticeable sign is often lolling of the head
Fails to react to parents	Failure to react in any way to a parent's face or voice. Abnormal reactions and apparent lack of recognition of a parent are also worrying signs
Possible sepsis	Suspected sepsis in patients who present with altered mental state, low blood pressure (systolic less than 100 mmHg) or raised respiratory rate (rate more than 22 breaths per minute) when using the qSOFA tool for assessment. Other sepsis screening tools may be used instead of qSOFA, and the relevant sepsis markers applied. In children, age-specific physiological tools should be used to determine if possibly septic
Persistent vomiting	Vomiting that is continuous or that occurs without any respite between episodes
Signs of dehydration	These include dry tongue, sunken eyes, decreased skin turgor and, in small babies, a sunken anterior fontanelle. Usually associated with a low urine output
Black or redcurrant stools	Any blackness fulfils the criteria of black stool while a dark red stool, classically seen in intussusceptions, is redcurrant stool
Jaundice	Neonatal jaundice
History of acutely vomiting blood	Frank haematemesis, vomiting of altered blood (coffee ground) or of blood mixed in the vomit within the past 24 hours
Vomiting	Any emesis

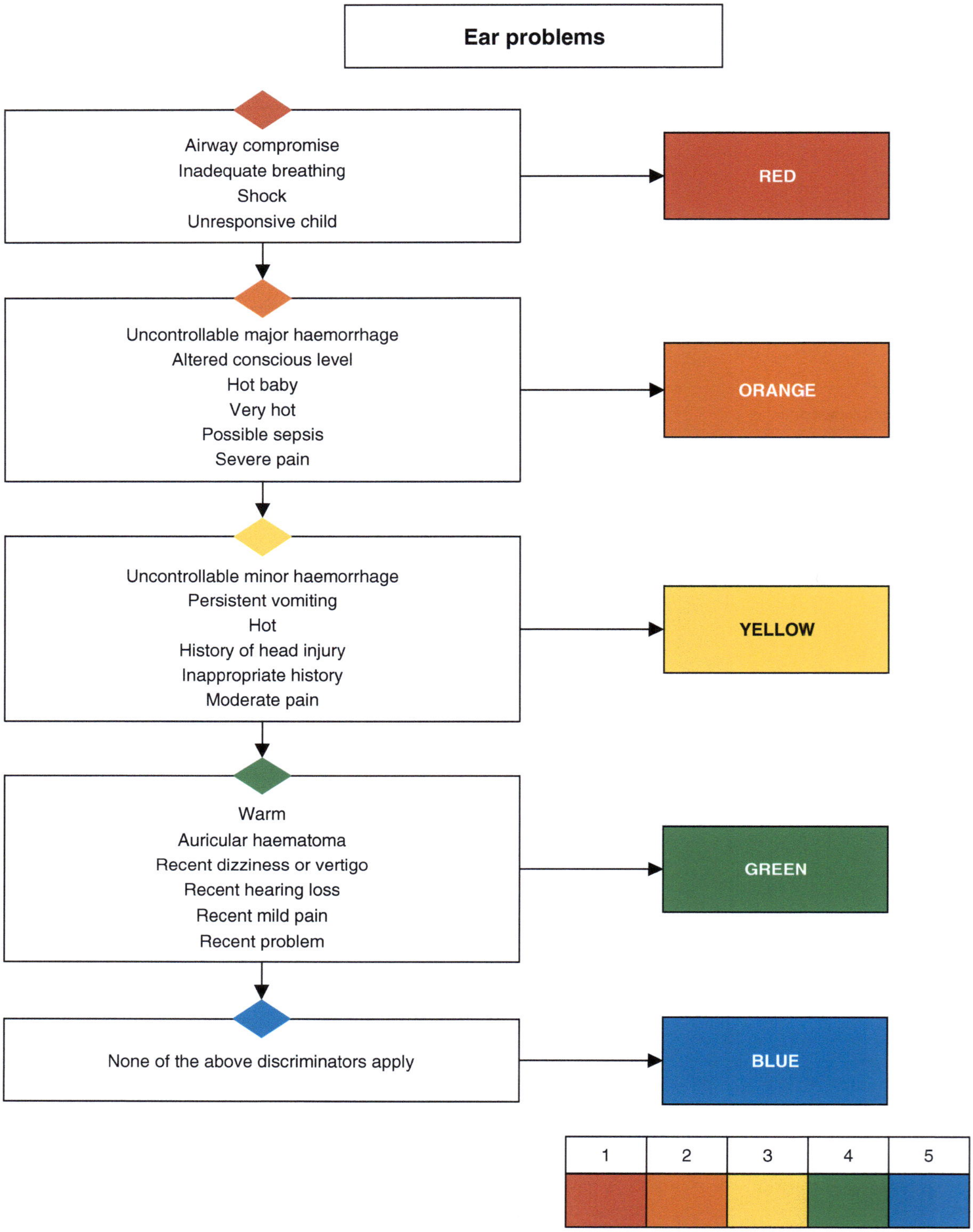
Ear problems
Airway compromise
Inadequate breathing
Shock
Unresponsive child
RED
Uncontrollable major haemorrhage
Altered conscious level
Hot baby
Very hot
Possible sepsis
Severe pain
ORANGE
Uncontrollable minor haemorrhage
Persistent vomiting
Hot
History of head injury
Inappropriate history
Moderate pain
YELLOW
Warm
Auricular haematoma
Recent dizziness or vertigo
Recent hearing loss
Recent mild pain
Recent problem
GREEN
None of the above discriminators apply
BLUE
1
2
3
4
5

Notes accompanying Ear problems

Related charts	Chart notes
Facial problems Head injury	This chart is designed to allow accurate prioritisation of patients presenting with conditions affecting the ear. A number of general discriminators are used including *Life threat*, *Pain*, *Haemorrhage* and *Temperature*

Relevant discriminators	Definition
Persistent vomiting	Vomiting that is continuous or that occurs without any respite between episodes
History of head injury	A history of a recent physically traumatic event involving the head. Usually this will be reported by the patient but if the patient has been unconscious this history should be sought from a reliable witness
Auricular haematoma	A tense haematoma (usually post traumatic) in the outer ear
Recent dizziness or vertigo	An acute feeling of spinning or dizziness, possibly accompanied by nausea and vomiting
Recent hearing loss	Loss of hearing in one or both ears within the previous week

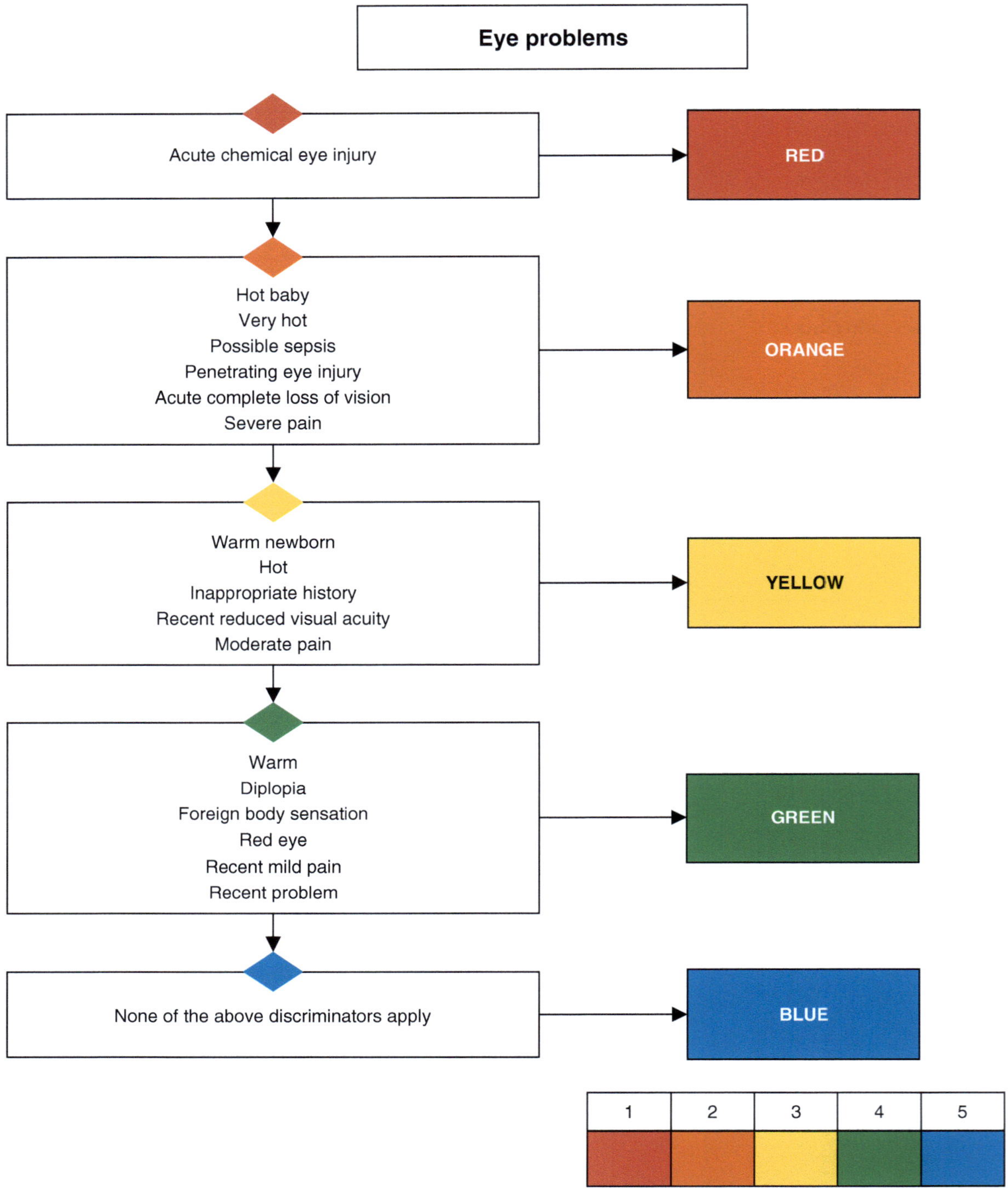
Eye problems
Acute chemical eye injury
RED
Hot baby
Very hot
Possible sepsis
Penetrating eye injury
Acute complete loss of vision
Severe pain
ORANGE
Warm newborn
Hot
Inappropriate history
Recent reduced visual acuity
Moderate pain
YELLOW
Warm
Diplopia
Foreign body sensation
Red eye
Recent mild pain
Recent problem
GREEN
None of the above discriminators apply
BLUE
1
2
3
4
5

Notes accompanying Eye problems

Related charts	Chart notes
Facial problems	This chart is designed to allow accurate prioritisation of patients attending with conditions affecting the eye. *Pain* is used as a general discriminator. A number of specific discriminators have been used including a history of *Acute chemical eye injury,* which indicates that immediate action is required, a history of *Penetrating eye injury* or sudden or *Acute complete loss of vision* and an assessment of visual acuity

Relevant discriminators	Definition
Acute chemical eye injury	Any substance splashed into or placed into the eye within the past 12 hours that caused stinging, burning or reduced vision should be assumed to have caused chemical injury
Possible sepsis	Suspected sepsis in patients who present with altered mental state, low blood pressure (systolic less than 100 mmHg) or raised respiratory rate (rate more than 22 breaths per minute) when using the qSOFA tool for assessment. Other sepsis screening tools may be used instead of qSOFA, and the relevant sepsis markers applied. In children, age-specific physiological tools should be used to determine if possibly septic
Penetrating eye injury	A recent physically traumatic event involving penetration of the globe
Acute complete loss of vision	Loss of vision in one or both eyes within the preceding 24 hours that has not returned to normal
Recent reduced visual acuity	Any reduction in corrected visual acuity within the past 7 days
Diplopia	Double vision that resolves when one eye is closed
Foreign body sensation	A sensation of something in the eye, often expressed as scraping or grittiness
Red eye	Any redness to the eye. A red eye may be painful or painless and may be complete or partial

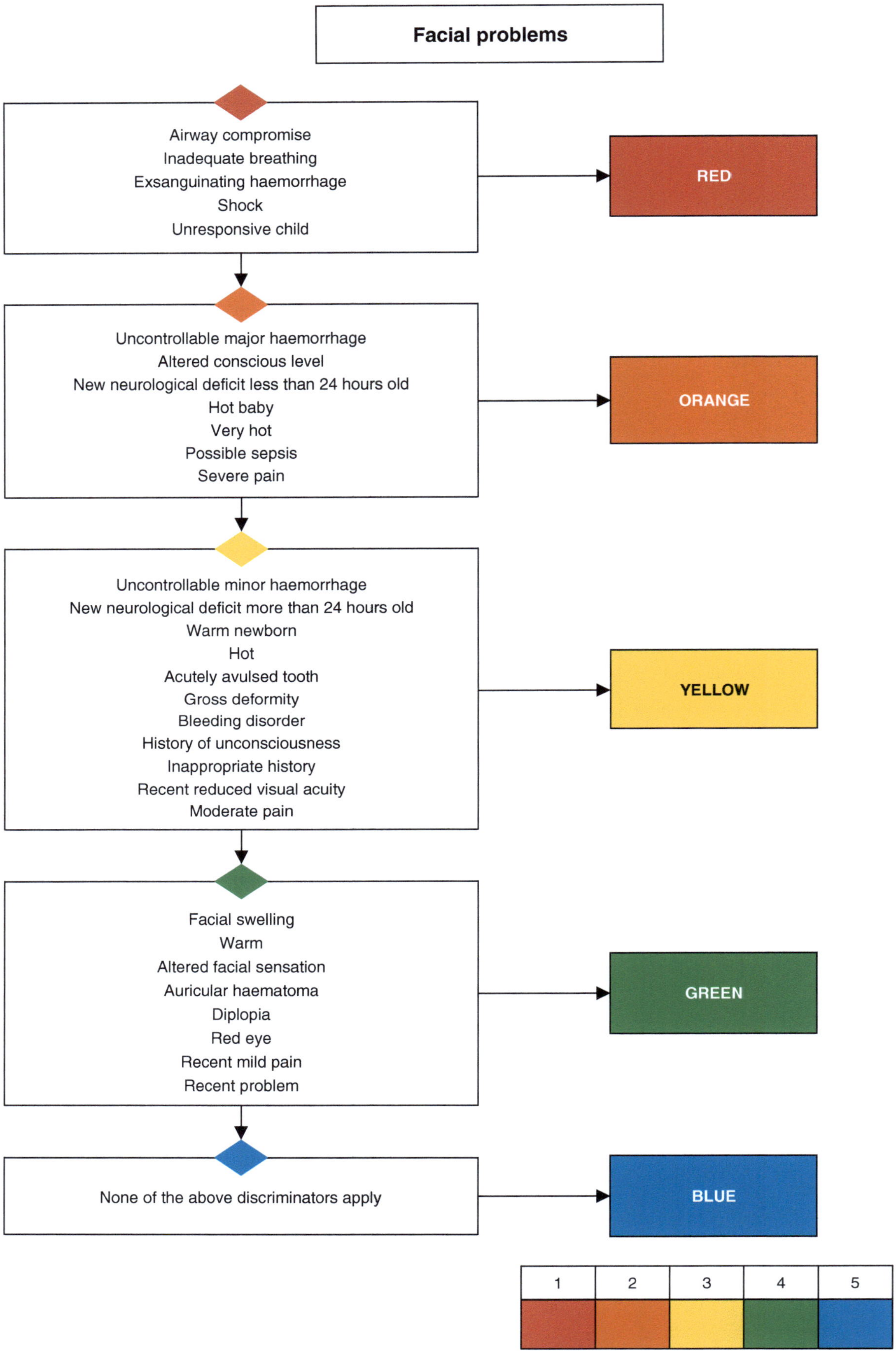
Facial problems
Airway compromise
Inadequate breathing
Exsanguinating haemorrhage
Shock
Unresponsive child
RED
Uncontrollable major haemorrhage
Altered conscious level
New neurological deficit less than 24 hours old
Hot baby
Very hot
Possible sepsis
Severe pain
ORANGE
Uncontrollable minor haemorrhage
New neurological deficit more than 24 hours old
Warm newborn
Hot
Acutely avulsed tooth
Gross deformity
Bleeding disorder
History of unconsciousness
Inappropriate history
Recent reduced visual acuity
Moderate pain
YELLOW
Facial swelling
Warm
Altered facial sensation
Auricular haematoma
Diplopia
Red eye
Recent mild pain
Recent problem
GREEN
None of the above discriminators apply
BLUE
1
2
3
4
5

Notes accompanying Facial problems

Related charts	Chart notes
Dental problems Ear problems Eye problems Head injury	This chart is designed to allow accurate prioritisation of patients attending with problems affecting the face. A number of general discriminators have been used including *Life threat*, *Haemorrhage* and *Pain*

Relevant discriminators	Definition
New neurological deficit less than 24 hours old	Any loss of neurological function that has come on within the previous 24 hours. This might include altered or lost sensation, weakness of the limbs (either transiently or permanently) and alterations in bladder or bowel function
New neurological deficit more than 24 hours old	Any loss of neurological function including altered or lost sensation, weakness of the limbs (either transiently or permanently) and alterations in bladder or bowel function
Acutely avulsed tooth	A tooth that has been avulsed intact within the previous 24 hours
Gross deformity	This will always be subjective. Gross and abnormal angulation or rotation is implied
Bleeding disorder	Congenital or acquired bleeding disorder
Recent reduced visual acuity	Any reduction in corrected visual acuity within the past 7 days
Facial swelling	Swelling around the face which may be localised or diffuse
Altered facial sensation	Any alteration of sensation on the face
Auricular haematoma	A tense haematoma (usually post traumatic) in the outer ear
Diplopia	Double vision that resolves when one eye is closed
Red eye	Any redness to the eye. A red eye may be painful or painless and may be complete or partial

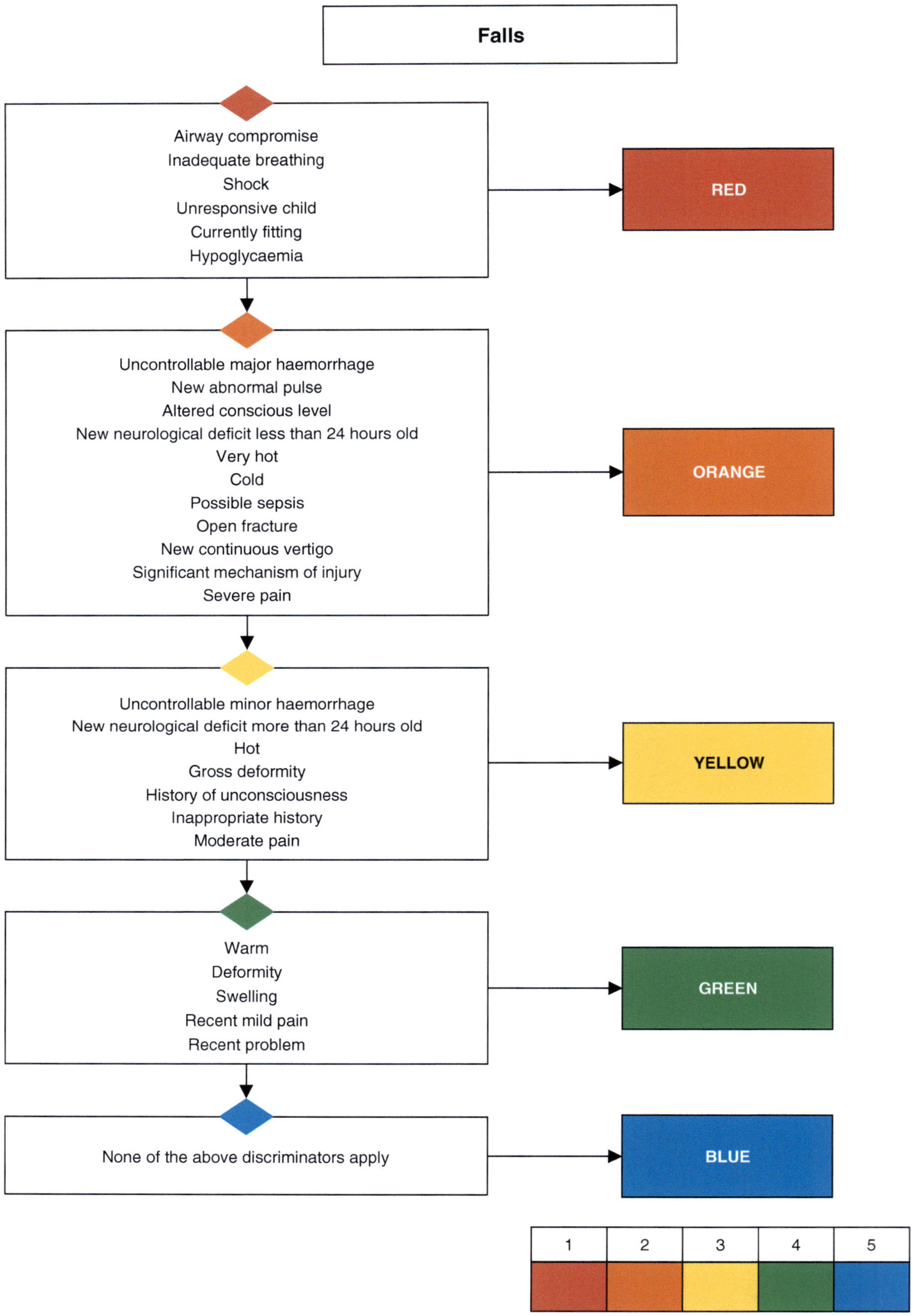
Falls
Airway compromise
Inadequate breathing
Shock
Unresponsive child
Currently fitting
Hypoglycaemia
RED
Uncontrollable major haemorrhage
New abnormal pulse
Altered conscious level
New neurological deficit less than 24 hours old
Very hot
Cold
Possible sepsis
Open fracture
New continuous vertigo
Significant mechanism of injury
Severe pain
ORANGE
Uncontrollable minor haemorrhage
New neurological deficit more than 24 hours old
Hot
Gross deformity
History of unconsciousness
Inappropriate history
Moderate pain
YELLOW
Warm
Deformity
Swelling
Recent mild pain
Recent problem
GREEN
None of the above discriminators apply
BLUE
1
2
3
4
5

Notes accompanying Falls

Related charts	Chart notes
Collapse	Many patients who present with a history of falls have suffered trauma as a result, and their priority will reflect the injuries suffered. Some, however, may have had a serious underlying pathology that caused them to fall, or may have developed complications after falling. This chart is designed to allow accurate prioritisation whether the injury or underlying cause is more pressing. A number of general discriminators have been included to ensure that patients suffering from serious underlying conditions or limb-threatening injuries are given a high priority

Relevant discriminators	Definition
Hypoglycaemia	Glucose less than 3 mmol/l
New neurological deficit less than 24 hours old	Any loss of neurological function that has come on within the previous 24 hours. This might include altered or lost sensation, weakness of the limbs (either transiently or permanently) and alterations in bladder or bowel function
Possible sepsis	Suspected sepsis in patients who present with altered mental state, low blood pressure (systolic less than 100 mmHg) or raised respiratory rate (rate more than 22 breaths per minute) when using the qSOFA tool for assessment. Other sepsis screening tools may be used instead of qSOFA, and the relevant sepsis markers applied. In children, age-specific physiological tools should be used to determine if possibly septic
Open fracture	All wounds in the vicinity of a fracture should be regarded with suspicion. If there is any possibility of communication between the wound and the fracture then the fracture should be assumed to be open
New continuous vertigo	New sensation of dizziness or vertigo which is continuous, and which has started within the previous 24 hours
Significant mechanism of injury	Penetrating injuries (stab or gunshot) and injuries with high energy transfer. In the frail/elderly, low energy transfer such as a fall from standing may be significant
New neurological deficit more than 24 hours old	Any loss of neurological function including altered or lost sensation, weakness of the limbs (either transiently or permanently) and alterations in bladder or bowel function
Gross deformity	This will always be subjective. Gross and abnormal angulation or rotation is implied
Inappropriate history	When the history (story) given does not explain the physical findings it is termed inappropriate. This is important as it is a marker of safeguarding concerns in both adults and children
Deformity	This will always be subjective. Abnormal angulation or rotation is implied
Swelling	An abnormal increase in size

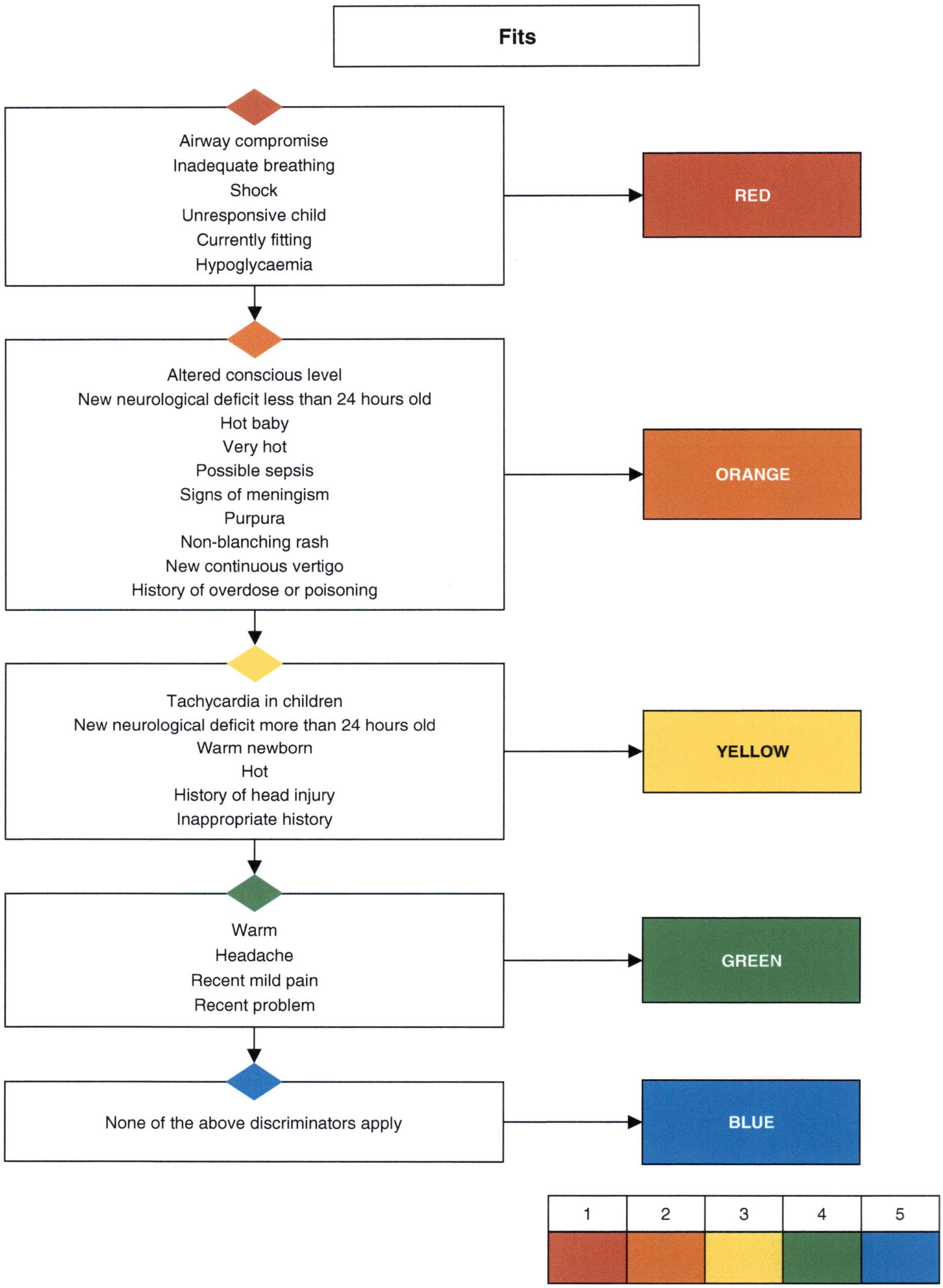
Fits
Airway compromise
Inadequate breathing
Shock
Unresponsive child
Currently fitting
Hypoglycaemia
RED
Altered conscious level
New neurological deficit less than 24 hours old
Hot baby
Very hot
Possible sepsis
Signs of meningism
Purpura
Non-blanching rash
New continuous vertigo
History of overdose or poisoning
ORANGE
Tachycardia in children
New neurological deficit more than 24 hours old
Warm newborn
Hot
History of head injury
Inappropriate history
YELLOW
Warm
Headache
Recent mild pain
Recent problem
GREEN
None of the above discriminators apply
BLUE
1
2
3
4
5

Notes accompanying Fits

Related charts	Chart notes
Head injury Headache Overdose and poisoning	Fitting is not an uncommon presentation to urgent and emergency care, and this chart is designed to allow rapid categorisation of patients who are currently fitting or who have fitted. A number of general discriminators are used including *Life threat*, *Conscious level* and *Temperature*. Specific discriminators include *Signs of meningism* and a focal or progressive loss of function. As with all unconscious patients, rapid blood sugar estimation would be indicated to exclude hypoglycaemia

Relevant discriminators	Definition
Hypoglycaemia	Glucose less than 3 mmol/l
New neurological deficit less than 24 hours old	Any loss of neurological function that has come on within the previous 24 hours. This might include altered or lost sensation, weakness of the limbs (either transiently or permanently) and alterations in bladder or bowel function
Possible sepsis	Suspected sepsis in patients who present with altered mental state, low blood pressure (systolic less than 100 mmHg) or raised respiratory rate (rate more than 22 breaths per minute) when using the qSOFA tool for assessment. Other sepsis screening tools may be used instead of qSOFA, and the relevant sepsis markers applied. In children, age-specific physiological tools should be used to determine if possibly septic
Signs of meningism	Classically, a stiff neck together with headache and photophobia
Purpura	A rash on any part of the body that is caused by small haemorrhages under the skin. A purpuric rash does not blanch (go white) when pressure is applied to it
Non-blanching rash	A rash that does not blanch (go white) when pressure is applied to it. Often tested using a glass tumbler to apply pressure as any colour change can be observed through the bottom of the tumbler
New continuous vertigo	New sensation of dizziness or vertigo which is continuous, and which has started within the previous 24 hours
History of overdose or poisoning	This information may come from others or may be deduced if medication is missing
Tachycardia in children	A child less than 1 year with a heart rate of 160 bpm or above ***OR*** a child 1 year or above with a heart rate of 140 bpm or above
New neurological deficit more than 24 hours old	Any loss of neurological function including altered or lost sensation, weakness of the limbs (either transiently or permanently) and alterations in bladder or bowel function
History of head injury	A history of a recent physically traumatic event involving the head. Usually this will be reported by the patient but if the patient has been unconscious this history should be sought from a reliable witness
Headache	Any pain around the head that is not related to a particular anatomical structure. Facial pain is not included

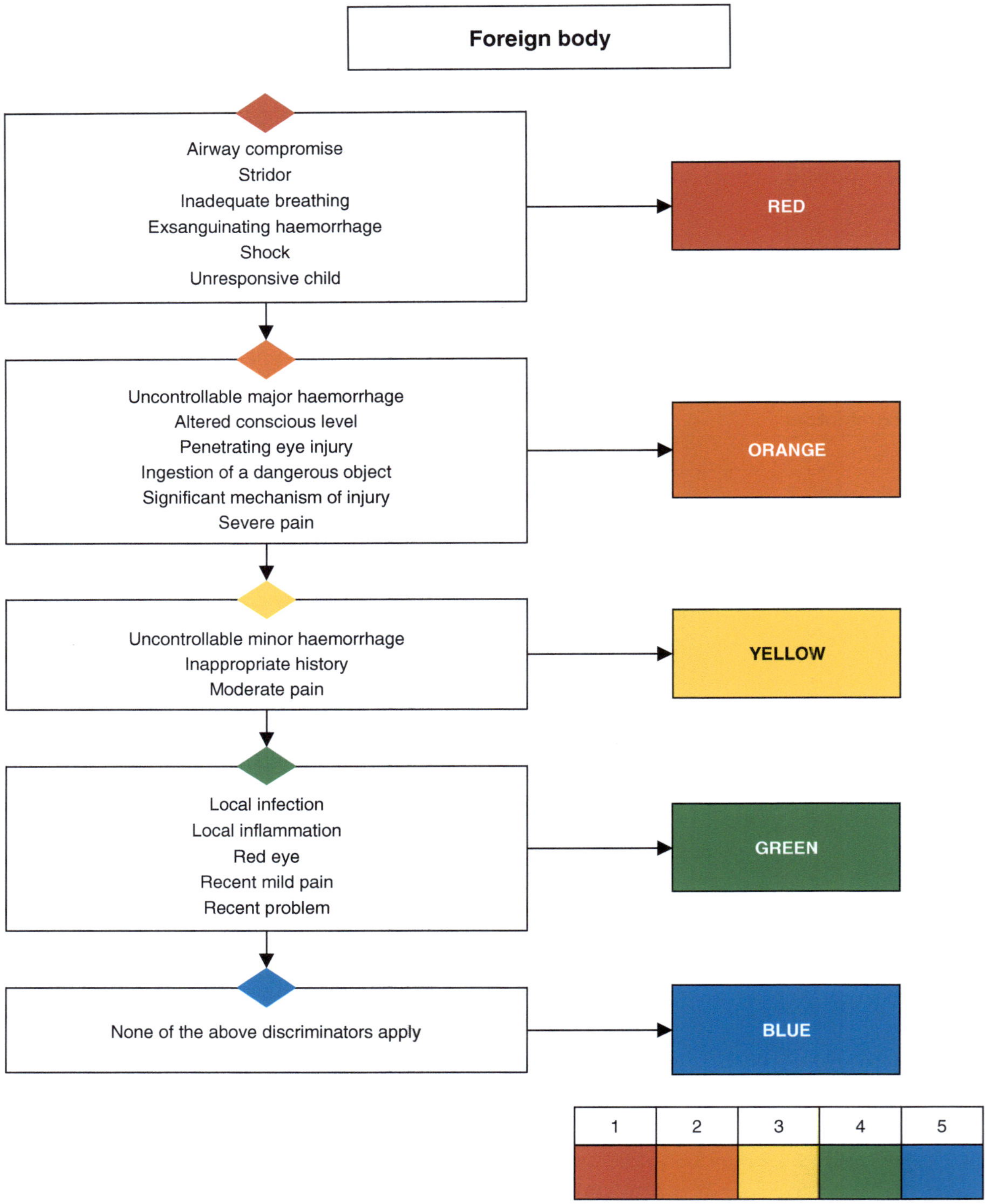
Foreign body
Airway compromise
Stridor
Inadequate breathing
Exsanguinating haemorrhage
Shock
Unresponsive child
RED
Uncontrollable major haemorrhage
Altered conscious level
Penetrating eye injury
Ingestion of a dangerous object
Significant mechanism of injury
Severe pain
ORANGE
Uncontrollable minor haemorrhage
Inappropriate history
Moderate pain
YELLOW
Local infection
Local inflammation
Red eye
Recent mild pain
Recent problem
GREEN
None of the above discriminators apply
BLUE
1
2
3
4
5

Notes accompanying Foreign body

Related charts	Chart notes
Wounds	This chart is designed to allow accurate prioritisation of patients who present with foreign bodies in any part of their anatomy. The severity of such cases can range from the inconvenient to the life threatening and this chart is designed to differentiate between these. A number of general discriminators have been used including *Life threat*, *Haemorrhage* and *Pain*. The only specific discriminator that relates to anatomical site is that of *Penetrating eye injury*

Relevant discriminators	Definition
Stridor	This may be an inspiratory or expiratory noise, or both. Stridor is heard best on breathing with the mouth open
Penetrating eye injury	A recent physically traumatic event involving penetration of the globe
Ingestion of a dangerous object	Ingestion of a dangerous or potentially dangerous foreign object, e.g. button battery, magnets or razor blades, which may be a potential threat to life
Significant mechanism of injury	Penetrating injuries (stab or gunshot) and injuries with high energy transfer. In the frail/elderly, low energy transfer such as a fall from standing may be significant
Inappropriate history	When the history (story) given does not explain the physical findings it is termed inappropriate. This is important as it is a marker of safeguarding concerns in both adults and children
Local infection	Local infection usually manifests as inflammation (pain, swelling and redness) confined to a particular site or area, with or without a collection of pus
Local inflammation	Local inflammation will involve pain, swelling and redness confined to a particular site or area
Red eye	Any redness to the eye. A red eye may be painful or painless and may be complete or partial

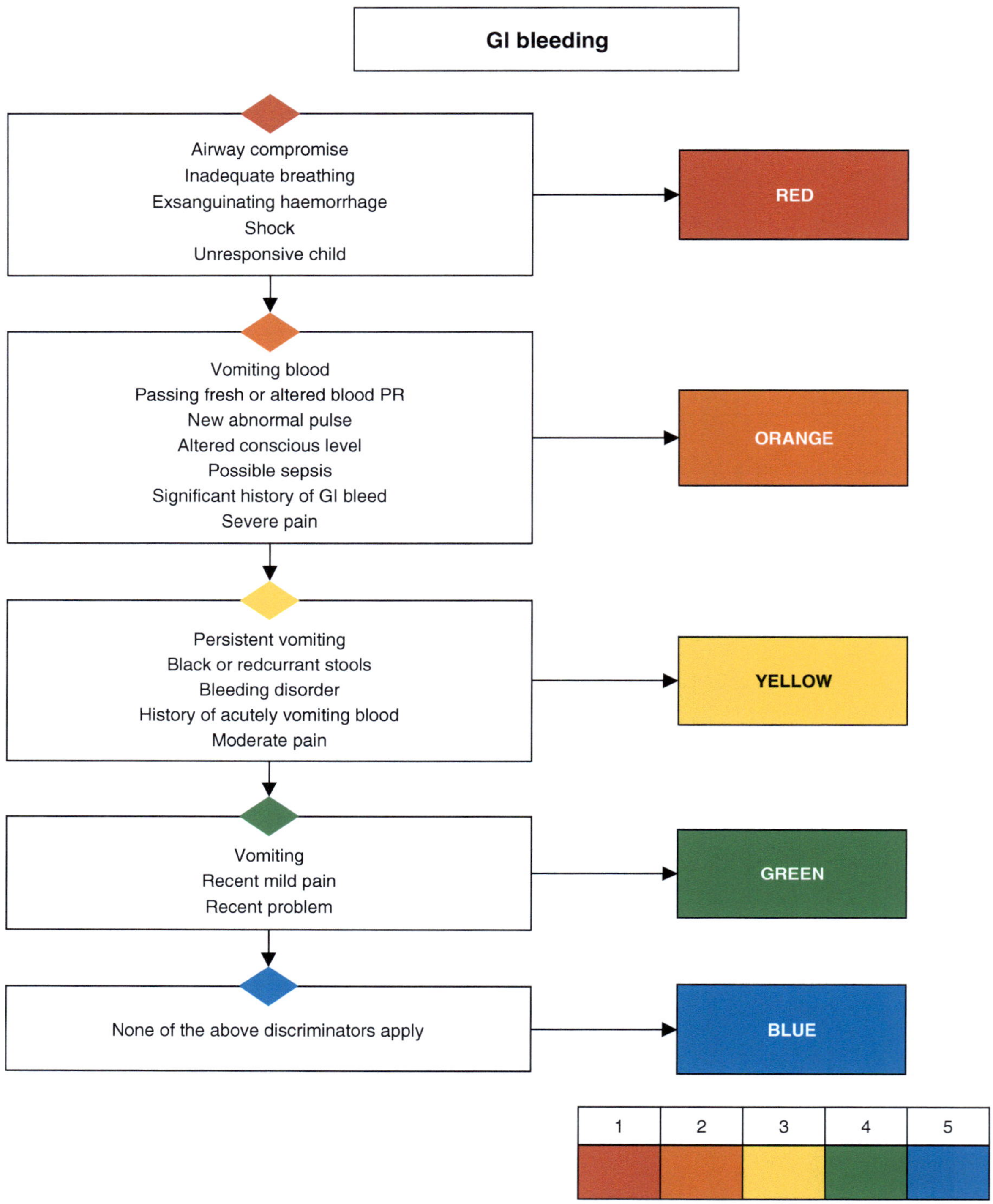
GI bleeding
Airway compromise
Inadequate breathing
Exsanguinating haemorrhage
Shock
Unresponsive child
RED
Vomiting blood
Passing fresh or altered blood PR
New abnormal pulse
Altered conscious level
Possible sepsis
Significant history of GI bleed
Severe pain
ORANGE
Persistent vomiting
Black or redcurrant stools
Bleeding disorder
History of acutely vomiting blood
Moderate pain
YELLOW
Vomiting
Recent mild pain
Recent problem
GREEN
None of the above discriminators apply
BLUE
1
2
3
4
5

Notes accompanying GI bleeding

Related charts	Chart notes
Abdominal pain in adults Abdominal pain in children Diarrhoea and vomiting in adults Diarrhoea and vomiting in children	Patients may present with GI bleeding either as vomiting altered or unaltered blood, or by passing blood PR. A number of general discriminators are used including *Life threat* and *Pain*. Specific discriminators have been selected to indicate the current severity of the GI bleeding. Thus patients vomiting blood or those passing fresh or altered blood PR have a higher category than those with a history of vomiting

Relevant discriminators	Definition
Vomiting blood	Vomited blood may be fresh (bright or dark red) or coffee ground in appearance
Passing fresh or altered blood PR	In active massive GI bleeding, dark red blood will be passed PR. As GI transit time increases this becomes darker, eventually becoming melaena
Possible sepsis	Suspected sepsis in patients who present with altered mental state, low blood pressure (systolic less than 100 mmHg) or raised respiratory rate (rate more than 22 breaths per minute) when using the qSOFA tool for assessment. Other sepsis screening tools may be used instead of qSOFA, and the relevant sepsis markers applied. In children, age-specific physiological tools should be used to determine if possibly septic
Significant history of GI bleed	Any history of massive GI bleeding or of any GI bleeding associated with oesophageal varices
Persistent vomiting	Vomiting that is continuous or that occurs without any respite between episodes
Black or redcurrant stools	Any blackness fulfils the criteria of black stool while a dark red stool, classically seen in intussusceptions, is redcurrant stool
Bleeding disorder	Congenital or acquired bleeding disorder
History of acutely vomiting blood	Frank haematemesis, vomiting of altered blood (coffee ground) or of blood mixed in the vomit within the past 24 hours
Vomiting	Any emesis

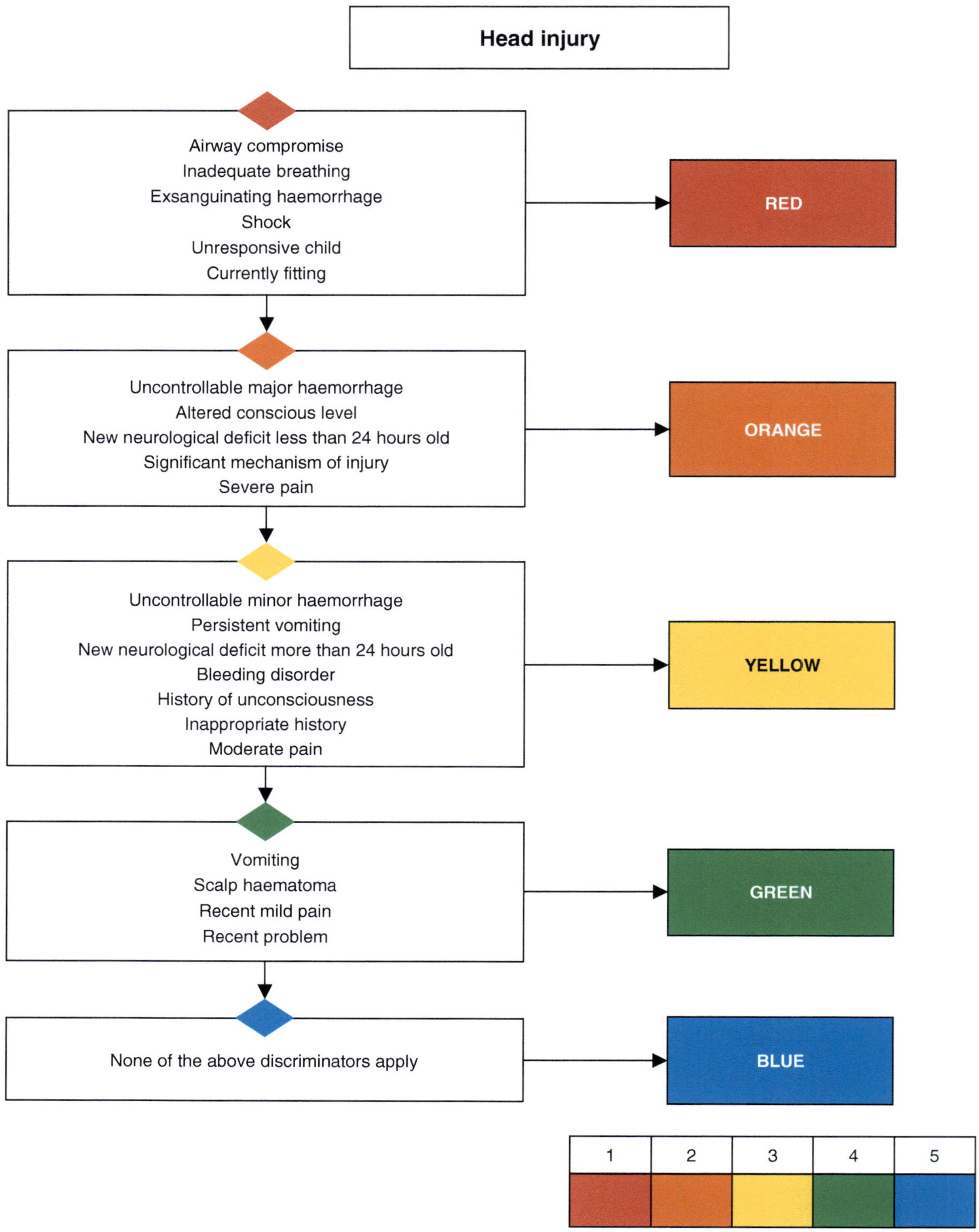
Head injury
Airway compromise
Inadequate breathing
Exsanguinating haemorrhage
Shock
Unresponsive child
Currently fitting
RED
Uncontrollable major haemorrhage
Altered conscious level
New neurological deficit less than 24 hours old
Significant mechanism of injury
Severe pain
ORANGE
Uncontrollable minor haemorrhage
Persistent vomiting
New neurological deficit more than 24 hours old
Bleeding disorder
History of unconsciousness
Inappropriate history
Moderate pain
YELLOW
Vomiting
Scalp haematoma
Recent mild pain
Recent problem
GREEN
None of the above discriminators apply
BLUE
1
2
3
4
5

Notes accompanying Head injury

Related charts	**Chart notes**
Fits Headache Neck pain	Head injury is an extremely common presentation and its effects may vary from life-threatening extradural haemorrhage to minimal scalp injury. A number of general discriminators have been used including *Life threat*, *Conscious level (in adults and children)*, *Haemorrhage* and *Pain*. Specific discriminators are included to select those patients with a significant mechanism and the development of neurological signs and symptoms to a higher priority

Relevant discriminators	**Definition**
New neurological deficit less than 24 hours old	Any loss of neurological function that has come on within the previous 24 hours. This might include altered or lost sensation, weakness of the limbs (either transiently or permanently) and alterations in bladder or bowel function
Significant mechanism of injury	Penetrating injuries (stab or gunshot) and injuries with high energy transfer. In the frail/elderly, low energy transfer such as a fall from standing may be significant
Persistent vomiting	Vomiting that is continuous or that occurs without any respite between episodes
New neurological deficit more than 24 hours old	Any loss of neurological function including altered or lost sensation, weakness of the limbs (either transiently or permanently) and alterations in bladder or bowel function
Bleeding disorder	Congenital or acquired bleeding disorder
Inappropriate history	When the history (story) given does not explain the physical findings it is termed inappropriate. This is important as it is a marker of safeguarding concerns in both adults and children
Vomiting	Any emesis
Scalp haematoma	A raised bruised area to the scalp (bruises below the hair line at the front are to the forehead)

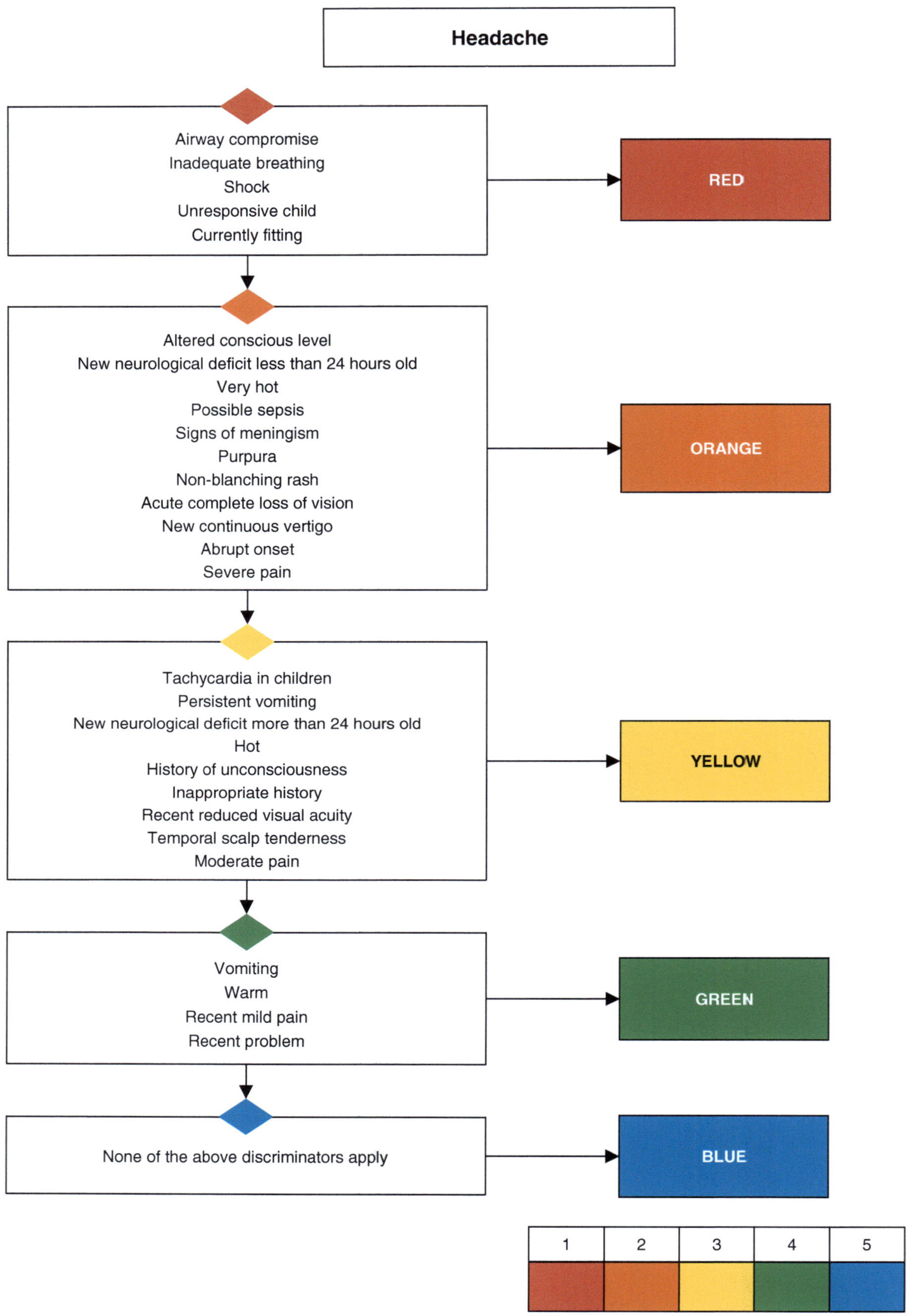
Headache
Airway compromise
Inadequate breathing
Shock
Unresponsive child
Currently fitting
RED
Altered conscious level
New neurological deficit less than 24 hours old
Very hot
Possible sepsis
Signs of meningism
Purpura
Non-blanching rash
Acute complete loss of vision
New continuous vertigo
Abrupt onset
Severe pain
ORANGE
Tachycardia in children
Persistent vomiting
New neurological deficit more than 24 hours old
Hot
History of unconsciousness
Inappropriate history
Recent reduced visual acuity
Temporal scalp tenderness
Moderate pain
YELLOW
Vomiting
Warm
Recent mild pain
Recent problem
GREEN
None of the above discriminators apply
BLUE
1
2
3
4
5

Notes accompanying Headache

Related charts	**Chart notes**
Head injury Neck pain	A large number of conditions can present with headache and a number of these require urgent intervention. A number of general discriminators are used including *Life threat*, *Conscious level*, *Pain* and *Temperature*. Specific discriminators have been used to identify severe causes such as subarachnoid haemorrhage and meningococcaemia. New neurological signs or symptoms together with reduction in visual acuity and tenderness of the scalp are used to indicate the need for urgent clinical review

Relevant discriminators	**Definition**
New neurological deficit less than 24 hours old	Any loss of neurological function that has come on within the previous 24 hours. This might include altered or lost sensation, weakness of the limbs (either transiently or permanently) and alterations in bladder or bowel function
Signs of meningism	Classically a stiff neck together with headache and photophobia
Purpura	A rash on any part of the body that is caused by small haemorrhages under the skin. A purpuric rash does not blanch (go white) when pressure is applied to it
Non-blanching rash	A rash that does not blanch (go white) when pressure is applied to it. Often tested using a glass tumbler to apply pressure as any colour change can be observed through the bottom of the tumbler
Acute complete loss of vision	Loss of vision in one or both eyes within the preceding 24 hours that has not returned to normal
New continuous vertigo	New sensation of dizziness or vertigo which is continuous, and which has started within the previous 24 hours
Tachycardia in children	A child less than 1 year with a heart rate of 160 bpm or above ***OR*** a child 1 year or above with a heart rate of 140 bpm or above
Persistent vomiting	Vomiting that is continuous or that occurs without any respite between episodes
New neurological deficit more than 24 hours old	Any loss of neurological function including altered or lost sensation, weakness of the limbs (either transiently or permanently) and alterations in bladder or bowel function
Recent reduced visual acuity	Any reduction in corrected visual acuity within the past 7 days
Temporal scalp tenderness	Tenderness on palpation over the temporal area (especially over the artery)
Vomiting	Any emesis

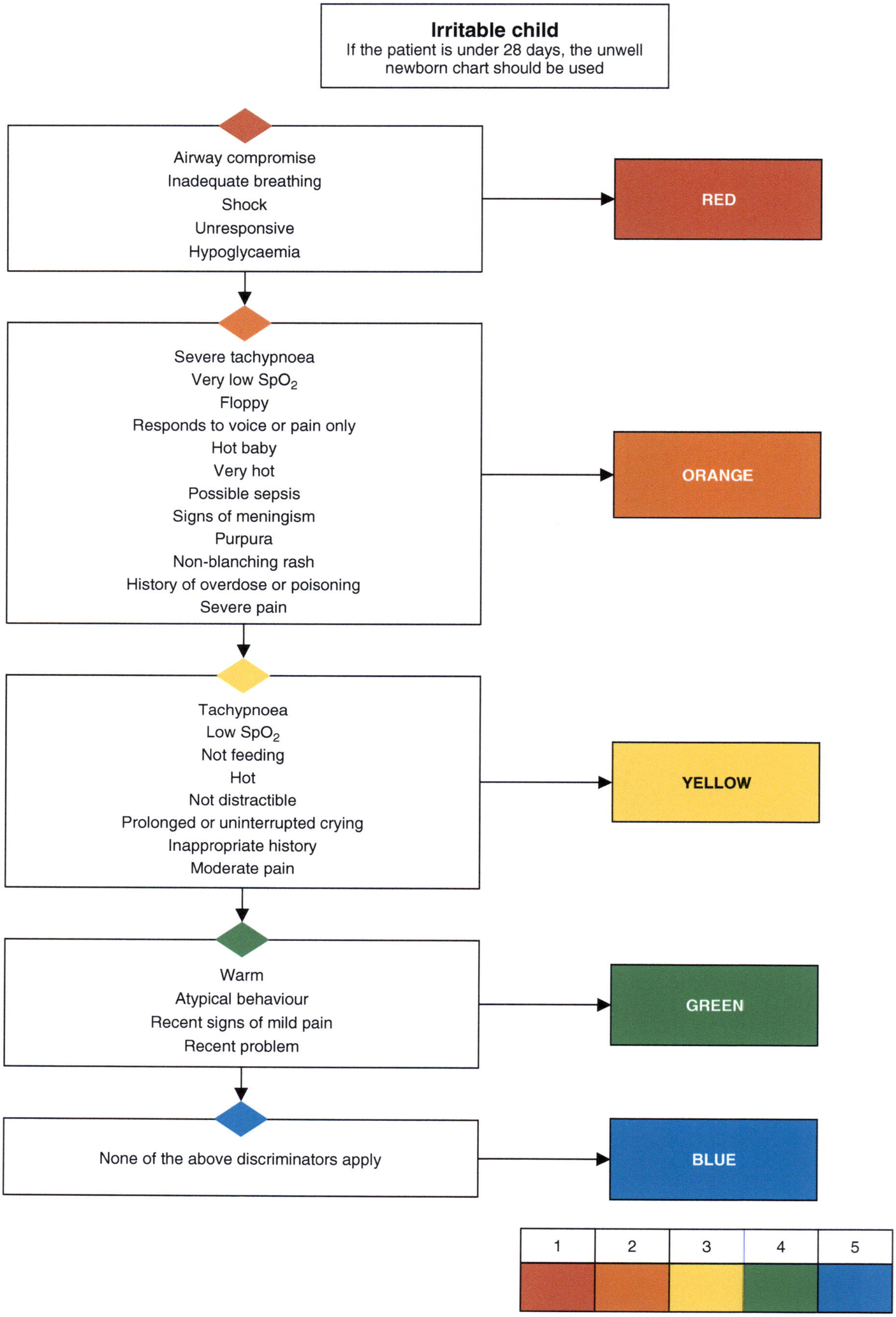
Irritable child
If the patient is under 28 days, the unwell newborn chart should be used
Airway compromise
Inadequate breathing
Shock
Unresponsive
Hypoglycaemia
RED
Severe tachypnoea
Very low SpO_2
Floppy
Responds to voice or pain only
Hot baby
Very hot
Possible sepsis
Signs of meningism
Purpura
Non-blanching rash
History of overdose or poisoning
Severe pain
ORANGE
Tachypnoea
Low SpO_2
Not feeding
Hot
Not distractible
Prolonged or uninterrupted crying
Inappropriate history
Moderate pain
YELLOW
Warm
Atypical behaviour
Recent signs of mild pain
Recent problem
GREEN
None of the above discriminators apply
BLUE
1
2
3
4
5

Notes accompanying Irritable child

Related charts	Chart notes
Crying baby Unwell baby Unwell child Unwell newborn Worried parent	This chart is designed to be used in children over the age of 12 months. A number of general discriminators have been used including *Life threat*, *Conscious level* and *Pain*. Specific discriminators include those that allow recognition of more specific pathologies such as septicaemia, or which indicate that a more serious pathology might exist. If the patient is under 28 days, the Unwell newborn chart should be used

Relevant discriminators	Definition
Hypoglycaemia	Glucose less than 3 mmol/l
Severe tachypnoea	A child less than 1 year with a respiratory rate of 55 breaths per minute or above ***OR*** a child 1 year or above with a respiratory rate of 45 breaths per minute or above
Floppy	Parents may describe their children as floppy. Tone is generally reduced – the most noticeable sign is often lolling of the head
Possible sepsis	Suspected sepsis in patients who present with altered mental state, low blood pressure (systolic less than 100 mmHg) or raised respiratory rate (rate more than 22 breaths per minute) when using the qSOFA tool for assessment. Other sepsis screening tools may be used instead of qSOFA, and the relevant sepsis markers applied. In children, age-specific physiological tools should be used to determine if possibly septic
Signs of meningism	Classically, a stiff neck together with headache and photophobia
Purpura	A rash on any part of the body that is caused by small haemorrhages under the skin. A purpuric rash does not blanch (go white) when pressure is applied to it
Non-blanching rash	A rash that does not blanch (go white) when pressure is applied to it. Often tested using a glass tumbler to apply pressure as any colour change can be observed through the bottom of the tumbler
Tachypnoea	A child less than 1 year with a respiratory rate of 45 breaths per minute or above ***OR*** a child 1 year or above with a respiratory rate of 35 breaths per minute or above
Not feeding	Children who will not take any solid or liquid (as appropriate) by mouth. Children who will take the food but always vomit afterwards may also fulfil this criterion
Not distractible	Children who are distressed by pain or other things who cannot be distracted by conversation or play
Prolonged or uninterrupted crying	A child who has cried continuously for 2 hours or more
Inappropriate history	When the history (story) given does not explain the physical findings it is termed inappropriate. This is important as it is a marker of safeguarding concerns in both adults and children
Atypical behaviour	Children who are behaving in a way that is not usual in the given situation. The carers will often volunteer this information. Such children are often referred to as fractious or 'out of sorts'

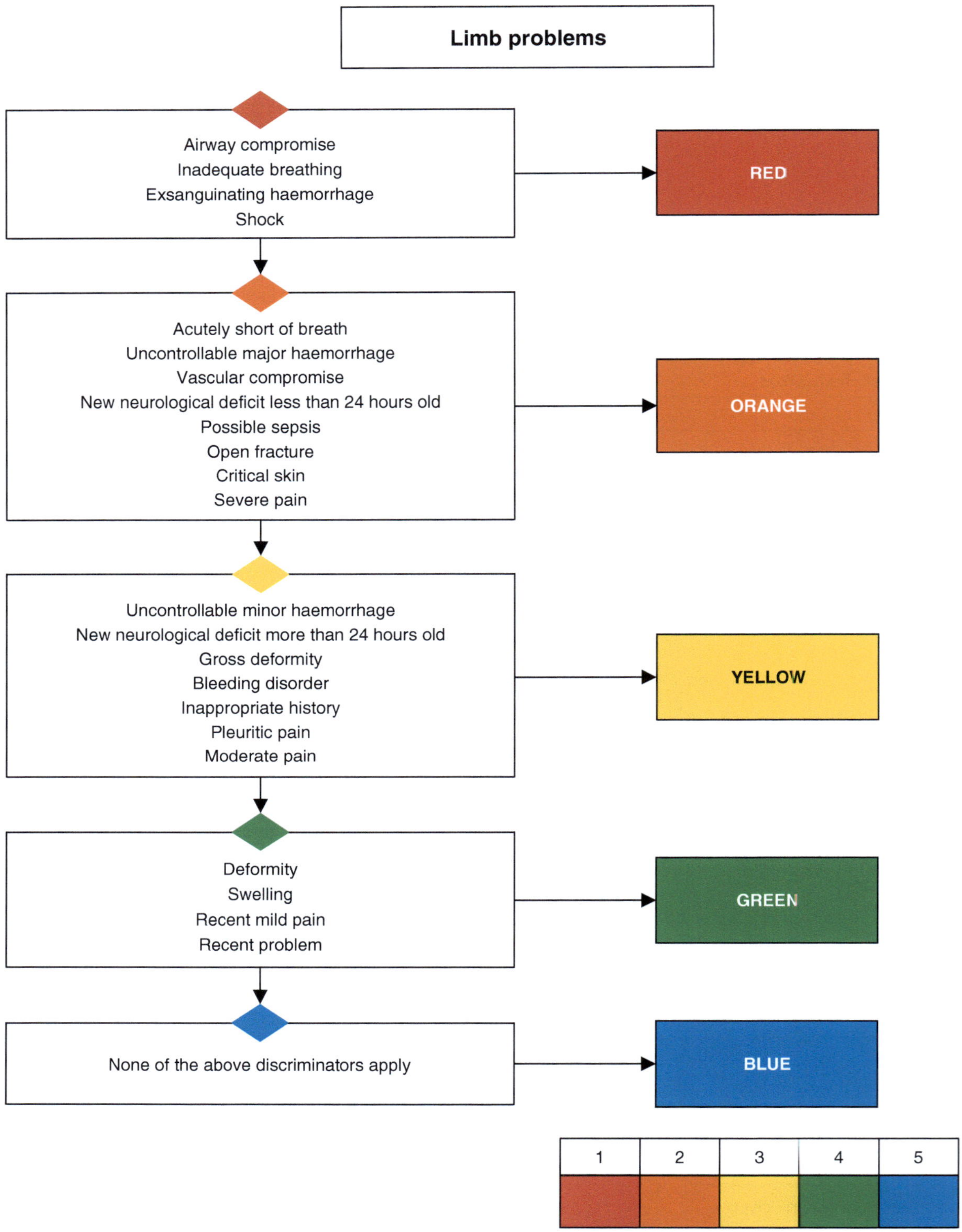
Limb problems
Airway compromise
Inadequate breathing
Exsanguinating haemorrhage
Shock
RED
Acutely short of breath
Uncontrollable major haemorrhage
Vascular compromise
New neurological deficit less than 24 hours old
Possible sepsis
Open fracture
Critical skin
Severe pain
ORANGE
Uncontrollable minor haemorrhage
New neurological deficit more than 24 hours old
Gross deformity
Bleeding disorder
Inappropriate history
Pleuritic pain
Moderate pain
YELLOW
Deformity
Swelling
Recent mild pain
Recent problem
GREEN
None of the above discriminators apply
BLUE
1
2
3
4
5

Notes accompanying Limb problems

Related charts	Chart notes
Limping child	Injuries to the limbs are the commonest presentation to urgent and emergency care departments, and, while rarely life-threatening, may cause considerable morbidity. A number of general discriminators are used including *Life threat*, *Haemorrhage* and *Pain*. Specific discriminators are included to ensure that limb-threatening injuries are seen and treated urgently. Discriminators are also included to remind the triage practitioner to consider the signs and symptoms of thromboembolic disease and its complications

Relevant discriminators	Definition
Vascular compromise	There will be a combination of pallor, coldness, altered sensation and pain with or without absent pulses distal to the injury
New neurological deficit less than 24 hours old	Any loss of neurological function that has come on within the previous 24 hours. This might include altered or lost sensation, weakness of the limbs (either transiently or permanently) and alterations in bladder or bowel function
Open fracture	All wounds in the vicinity of a fracture should be regarded with suspicion. If there is any possibility of communication between the wound and the fracture then the fracture should be assumed to be open
Critical skin	A fracture or dislocation may leave fragments or ends of bone pressing so hard against the skin that the viability of the skin is threatened. The skin will be white and under tension
New neurological deficit more than 24 hours old	Any loss of neurological function including altered or lost sensation, weakness of the limbs (either transiently or permanently) and alterations in bladder or bowel function
Gross deformity	This will always be subjective. Gross and abnormal angulation or rotation is implied
Bleeding disorder	Congenital or acquired bleeding disorder
Pleuritic pain	A sharp, localised pain in the chest that worsens on breathing, coughing or sneezing
Deformity	This will always be subjective. Abnormal angulation or rotation is implied
Swelling	An abnormal increase in size

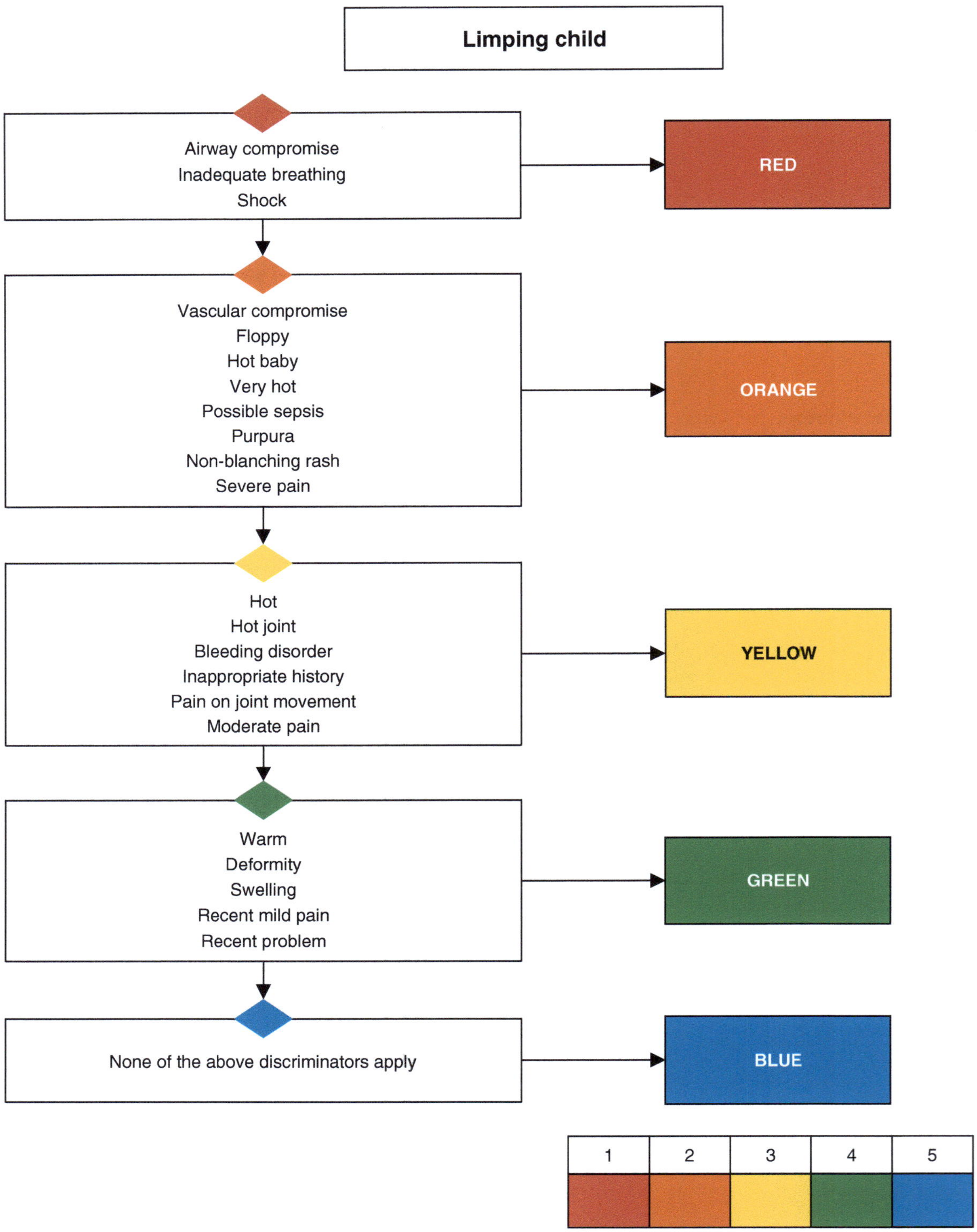
Limping child
Airway compromise
Inadequate breathing
Shock
RED
Vascular compromise
Floppy
Hot baby
Very hot
Possible sepsis
Purpura
Non-blanching rash
Severe pain
ORANGE
Hot
Hot joint
Bleeding disorder
Inappropriate history
Pain on joint movement
Moderate pain
YELLOW
Warm
Deformity
Swelling
Recent mild pain
Recent problem
GREEN
None of the above discriminators apply
BLUE
1
2
3
4
5

Notes accompanying Limping child

Related charts	Chart notes
Limb problems	Children who present with limp range from those who have suffered a minor soft tissue injury to the foot or ankle to those who have developed septic arthritis of the hip. This chart is designed to allow accurate prioritisation of such children. A number of general discriminators are used including *Life threat*, *Pain* and *Temperature*. Specific discriminators have been included to allow children with more urgent pathologies that threaten distal function to be accurately identified, and to spot quickly those in whom the limp is a sinister sign of systemic disease

Relevant discriminators	Definition
Vascular compromise	There will be a combination of pallor, coldness, altered sensation and pain with or without absent pulses distal to the injury
Possible sepsis	Suspected sepsis in patients who present with altered mental state, low blood pressure (systolic less than 100 mmHg) or raised respiratory rate (rate more than 22 breaths per minute) when using the qSOFA tool for assessment. Other sepsis screening tools may be used instead of qSOFA, and the relevant sepsis markers applied. In children, age-specific physiological tools should be used to determine if possibly septic
Hot joint	Any warmth around a joint. Often accompanied by redness
Bleeding disorder	Congenital or acquired bleeding disorder
Pain on joint movement	This can be pain on either active (patient) movement or passive (examiner) movement
Deformity	This will always be subjective. Abnormal angulation or rotation is implied
Swelling	An abnormal increase in size

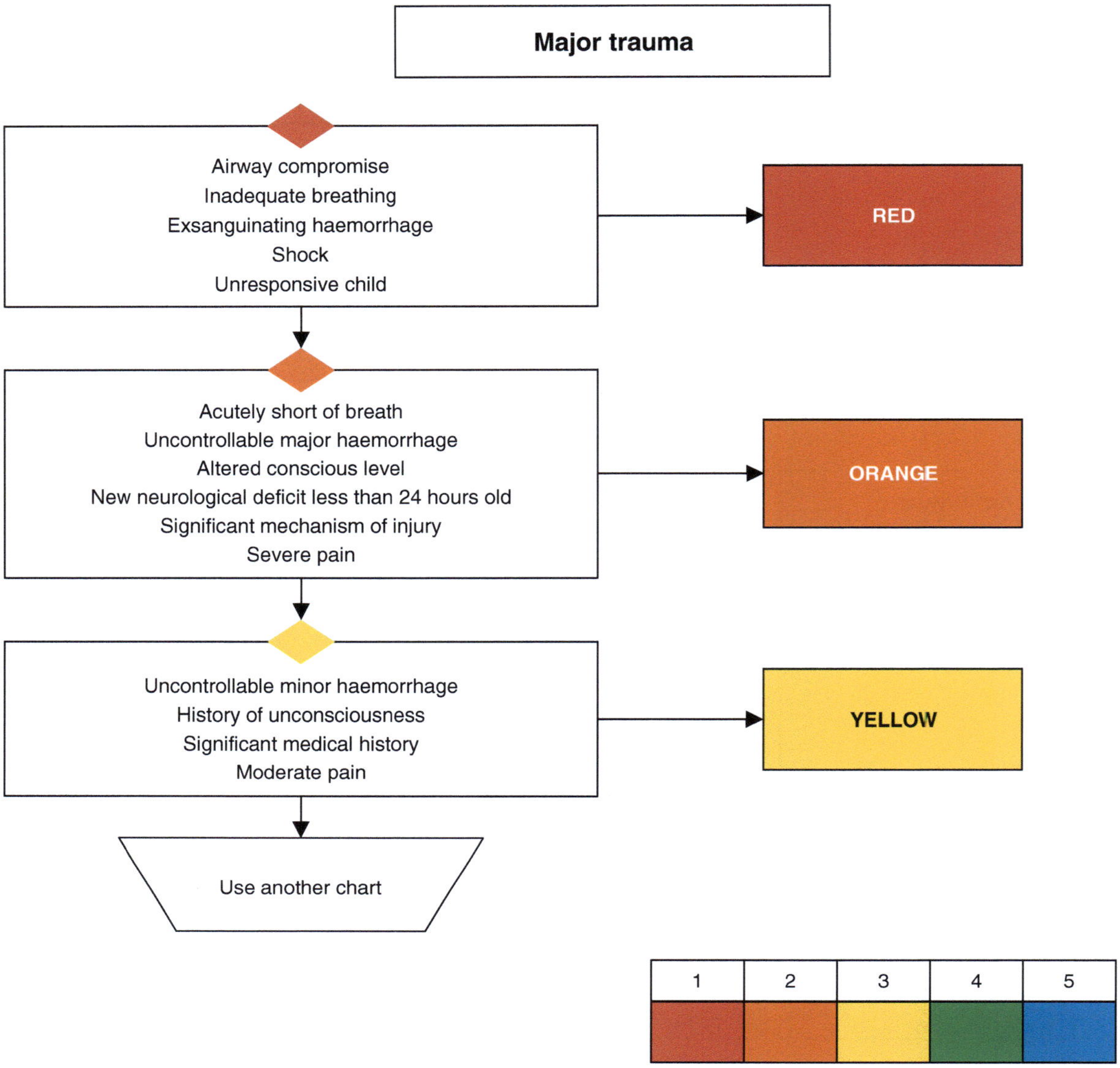
Major trauma
Airway compromise
Inadequate breathing
Exsanguinating haemorrhage
Shock
Unresponsive child
RED
Acutely short of breath
Uncontrollable major haemorrhage
Altered conscious level
New neurological deficit less than 24 hours old
Significant mechanism of injury
Severe pain
ORANGE
Uncontrollable minor haemorrhage
History of unconsciousness
Significant medical history
Moderate pain
YELLOW
Use another chart
1
2
3
4
5

Notes accompanying Major trauma

Related charts	Chart notes
None	Most healthcare providers know what is implied by major trauma but it is a strange presentation in that it is defined not by the patients or their injuries, but on some judgement of that injury by the carers. For this reason it is impossible to categorise a patient with this presentation as less than urgent. If it is necessary to do this, then a deliberate decision needs to be made that the original description of the patient as having suffered major trauma was incorrect, and the patient should be categorised using a different presentation flow diagram. A number of general discriminators have been used including *Life threat*, *Haemorrhage*, *Conscious level (both adult and child)* and *Pain*. Specific discriminators are designed to ensure that patients with a significant mechanism of injury are given a high enough urgency, and that those with pre-existing medical conditions and/or the development of new neurological signs are seen in good time

Relevant discriminators	Definition
Acutely short of breath	Shortness of breath that comes on suddenly, or a sudden exacerbation of chronic shortness of breath
New neurological deficit less than 24 hours old	Any loss of neurological function that has come on within the previous 24 hours. This might include altered or lost sensation, weakness of the limbs (either transiently or permanently) and alterations in bladder or bowel function
Significant mechanism of injury	Penetrating injuries (stab or gunshot) and injuries with high energy transfer. In the frail/elderly, low energy transfer such as a fall from standing may be significant
Significant medical history	Any pre-existing medical condition requiring continual medication or other care

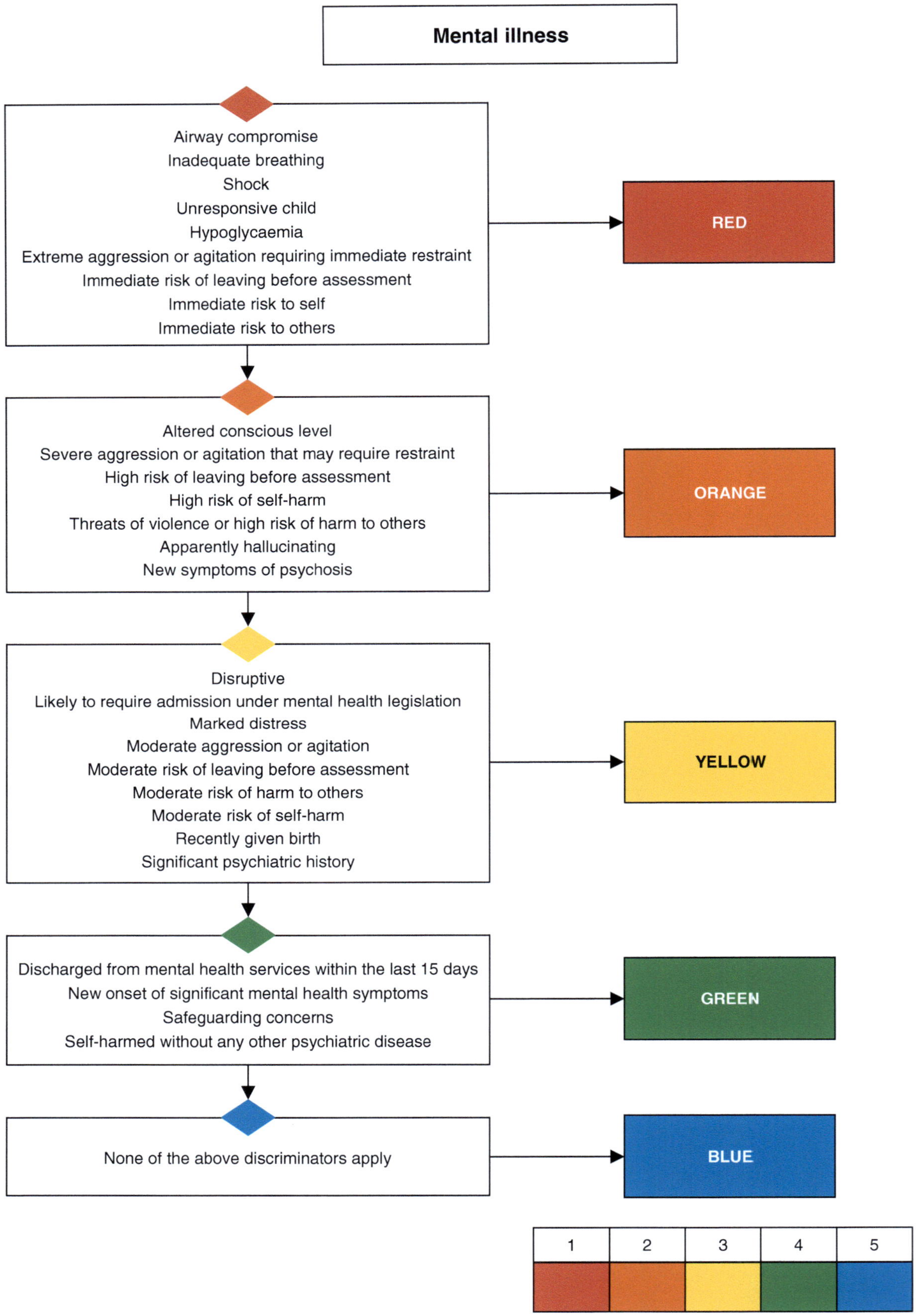
Mental illness
Airway compromise
Inadequate breathing
Shock
Unresponsive child
Hypoglycaemia
Extreme aggression or agitation requiring immediate restraint
Immediate risk of leaving before assessment
Immediate risk to self
Immediate risk to others
RED
Altered conscious level
Severe aggression or agitation that may require restraint
High risk of leaving before assessment
High risk of self-harm
Threats of violence or high risk of harm to others
Apparently hallucinating
New symptoms of psychosis
ORANGE
Disruptive
Likely to require admission under mental health legislation
Marked distress
Moderate aggression or agitation
Moderate risk of leaving before assessment
Moderate risk of harm to others
Moderate risk of self-harm
Recently given birth
Significant psychiatric history
YELLOW
Discharged from mental health services within the last 15 days
New onset of significant mental health symptoms
Safeguarding concerns
Self-harmed without any other psychiatric disease
GREEN
None of the above discriminators apply
BLUE
1
2
3
4
5

Notes accompanying Mental illness

Related charts	Chart notes
Apparently drunk Behaving strangely	This chart is designed to allow clinical prioritisation of patients who present with known or newly declared mental illness. This includes patients who attended with a chief complaint which would indicate mental illness. A number of general discriminators have been used including *Life threat* and *Conscious level*. This chart is designed to allow assessment of both physical and psychiatric aspects of the presentation. Specific discriminators are included to allow accurate prioritisation of patients with a known significant psychiatric history and those who have varying degrees of risk of causing harm to others or to themselves. Patients who are disruptive or who are suffering severe distress are placed in the urgent category

Relevant discriminators	Definition
Hypoglycaemia	Glucose less than 3 mmol/l
Extreme aggression or agitation requiring immediate restraint	Aggression and agitation of such a degree that immediate restraint is required to manage the risk of harm to self or others
Immediate risk of leaving before assessment	Active, credible attempts to leave prior to assessment pose an immediate risk
Immediate risk to self	An initial view of the risk of harm to self can be formed by considering the patient's behaviour. Patients who are actively harming themselves and those who are threatening to harm themselves and who have the means to do so are at immediate risk
Immediate risk to others	An initial view of the risk of harm to others can be judged by looking at posture (tense, clenched), speech (loud, using threatening words) and motor behaviour (restless, pacing, lunging at others). Immediate risk should be assumed if weapons and potential victims are available and no controls are already in place
Apparently hallucinating	Patients who are apparently hallucinating may appear distracted and may appear to react to stimuli (primarily visual and auditory) that are not apparent to anyone else
New symptoms of psychosis	Active new symptoms of psychosis with no insight such as hallucinations, delusions and/or paranoia
Likely to require admission under mental health legislation	Patients with significant psychiatric symptoms who are likely to require admission under mental health legislation
Recently given birth	A patient who has given birth within the past 3 months
Significant psychiatric history	A history of a major psychiatric illness or event
Discharged from mental health services within the last 15 days	Any patient who has been discharged from an active period of care under mental health services (in hospital or in the community) within the last 15 days
New onset of significant mental health symptoms	Any new mental health symptoms not already taken into account

Neck pain

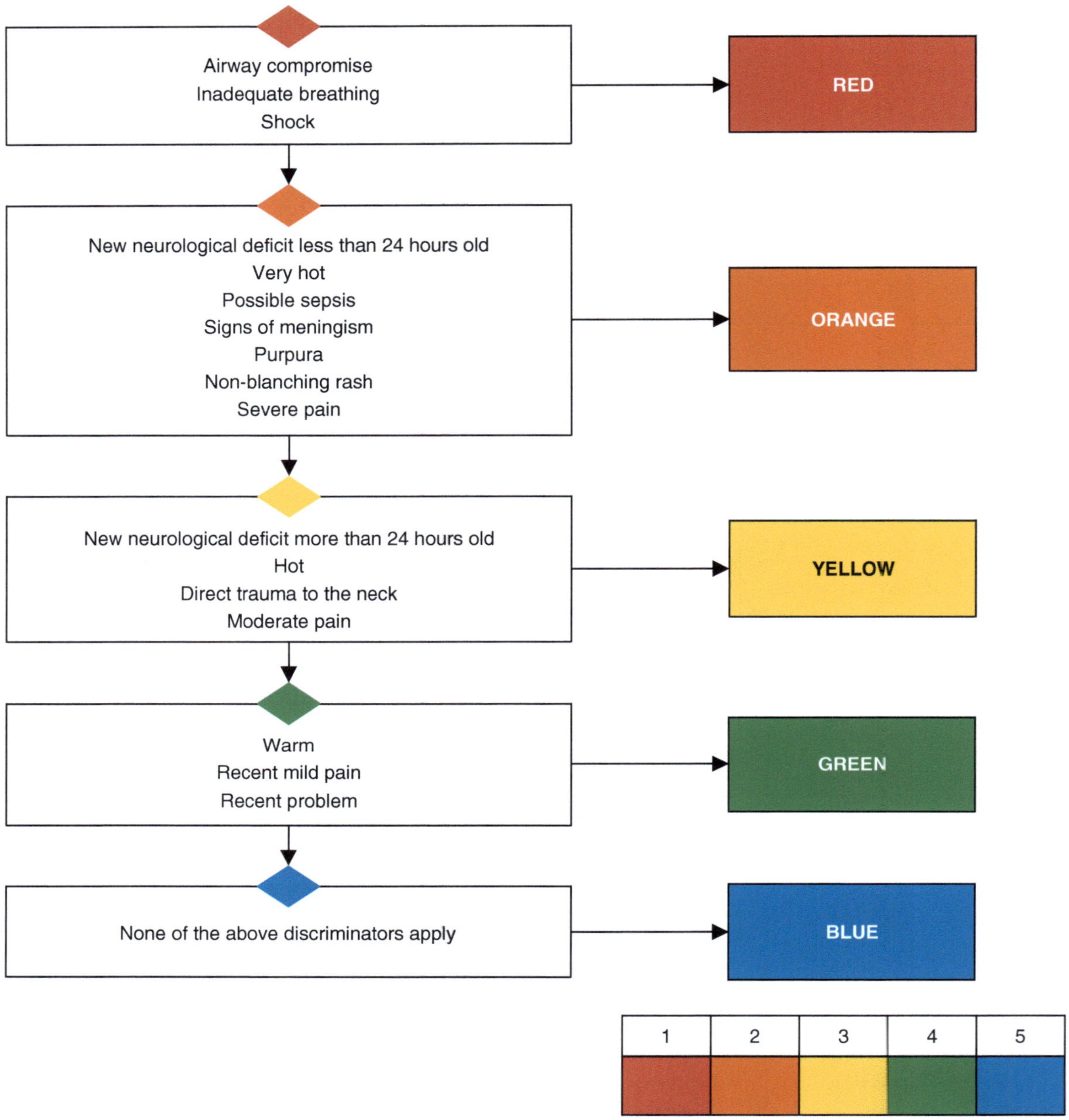
Airway compromise
Inadequate breathing
Shock
RED
New neurological deficit less than 24 hours old
Very hot
Possible sepsis
Signs of meningism
Purpura
Non-blanching rash
Severe pain
ORANGE
New neurological deficit more than 24 hours old
Hot
Direct trauma to the neck
Moderate pain
YELLOW
Warm
Recent mild pain
Recent problem
GREEN
None of the above discriminators apply
BLUE
1
2
3
4
5

Notes accompanying Neck pain

Related charts	Chart notes
Back pain Headache	Pain in the neck may arise because of local pathology or meningeal irritation. This chart is designed to allow rapid identification of patients presenting with symptoms or signs that indicate more urgent pathologies. A number of general discriminators are used including *Life threat*, *Pain* and *Temperature*. The specific discriminators that indicate meningitis are included under the ORANGE category

Relevant discriminators	Definition
New neurological deficit less than 24 hours old	Any loss of neurological function that has come on within the previous 24 hours. This might include altered or lost sensation, weakness of the limbs (either transiently or permanently) and alterations in bladder or bowel function
Possible sepsis	Suspected sepsis in patients who present with altered mental state, low blood pressure (systolic less than 100 mmHg) or raised respiratory rate (rate more than 22 breaths per minute) when using the qSOFA tool for assessment. Other sepsis screening tools may be used instead of qSOFA, and the relevant sepsis markers applied. In children, age-specific physiological tools should be used to determine if possibly septic
Signs of meningism	Classically, a stiff neck together with headache and photophobia
Purpura	A rash on any part of the body that is caused by small haemorrhages under the skin. A purpuric rash does not blanch (go white) when pressure is applied to it
Non-blanching rash	A rash that does not blanch (go white) when pressure is applied to it. Often tested using a glass tumbler to apply pressure as any colour change can be observed through the bottom of the tumbler
New neurological deficit more than 24 hours old	Any loss of neurological function including altered or lost sensation, weakness of the limbs (either transiently or permanently) and alterations in bladder or bowel function
Direct trauma to the neck	This may be top to bottom (loading), for instance when something falls on the head, bending (forwards, backwards or to the side) twisting or distracting such as hanging

Overdose and poisoning

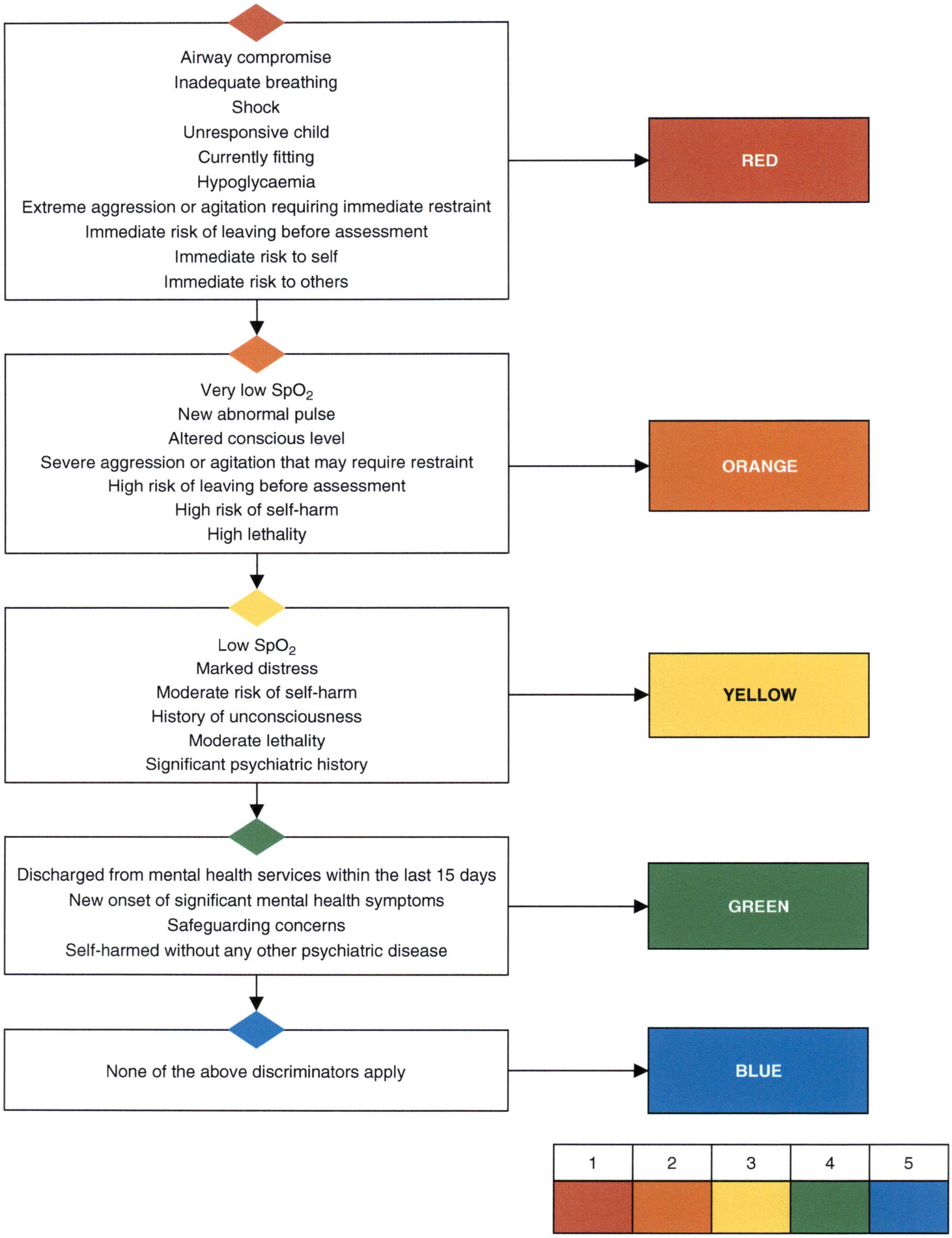

Notes accompanying Overdose and poisoning

Related charts	Chart notes
Self-harm	This flowchart is designed to allow both the physical and psychiatric aspects of overdose to be considered, and to ensure accurate prioritisation of patients from both perspectives. It also allows prioritisation of patients who have been accidentally (or deliberately) poisoned by others. A number of general discriminators have been used including *Life threat* and *Unconscious level (in adults and children)*. Specific discriminators include the assessed lethality of the overdose (which can be decided following discussion with a poisons centre) and an assessment of the risk of further attempts at self-harm

Relevant discriminators	Definition
Hypoglycaemia	Glucose less than 3 mmol/l
Extreme aggression or agitation requiring immediate restraint	Aggression and agitation of such a degree that immediate restraint is required to manage the risk of harm to self or others
Immediate risk of leaving before assessment	Active, credible attempts to leave prior to assessment pose an immediate risk
Immediate risk to self	An initial view of the risk of harm to self can be formed by considering the patient's behaviour. Patients who are actively harming themselves and those who are threatening to harm themselves and who have the means to do so are at immediate risk
Immediate risk to others	An initial view of the risk of harm to others can be judged by looking at posture (tense, clenched), speech (loud, using threatening words) and motor behaviour (restless, pacing, lunging at others). Immediate risk should be assumed if weapons and potential victims are available and no controls are already in place
High lethality	Lethality is the potential of the substance taken to cause harm. Advice from a poisons centre may be required to establish the level of risk of serious illness or death. If in doubt, assume a high risk
Marked distress	Patients who are markedly physically or emotionally upset
Moderate lethality	Lethality is the potential of the substance taken to cause serious illness or death. Advice from a poisons centre may be required to establish the level of risk to the patient
Significant psychiatric history	A history of a major psychiatric illness or event
Discharged from mental health services within the last 15 days	Any patient who has been discharged from an active period of care under mental health services (in hospital or in the community) within the last 15 days
New onset of significant mental health symptoms	Any new mental health symptoms not already taken into account

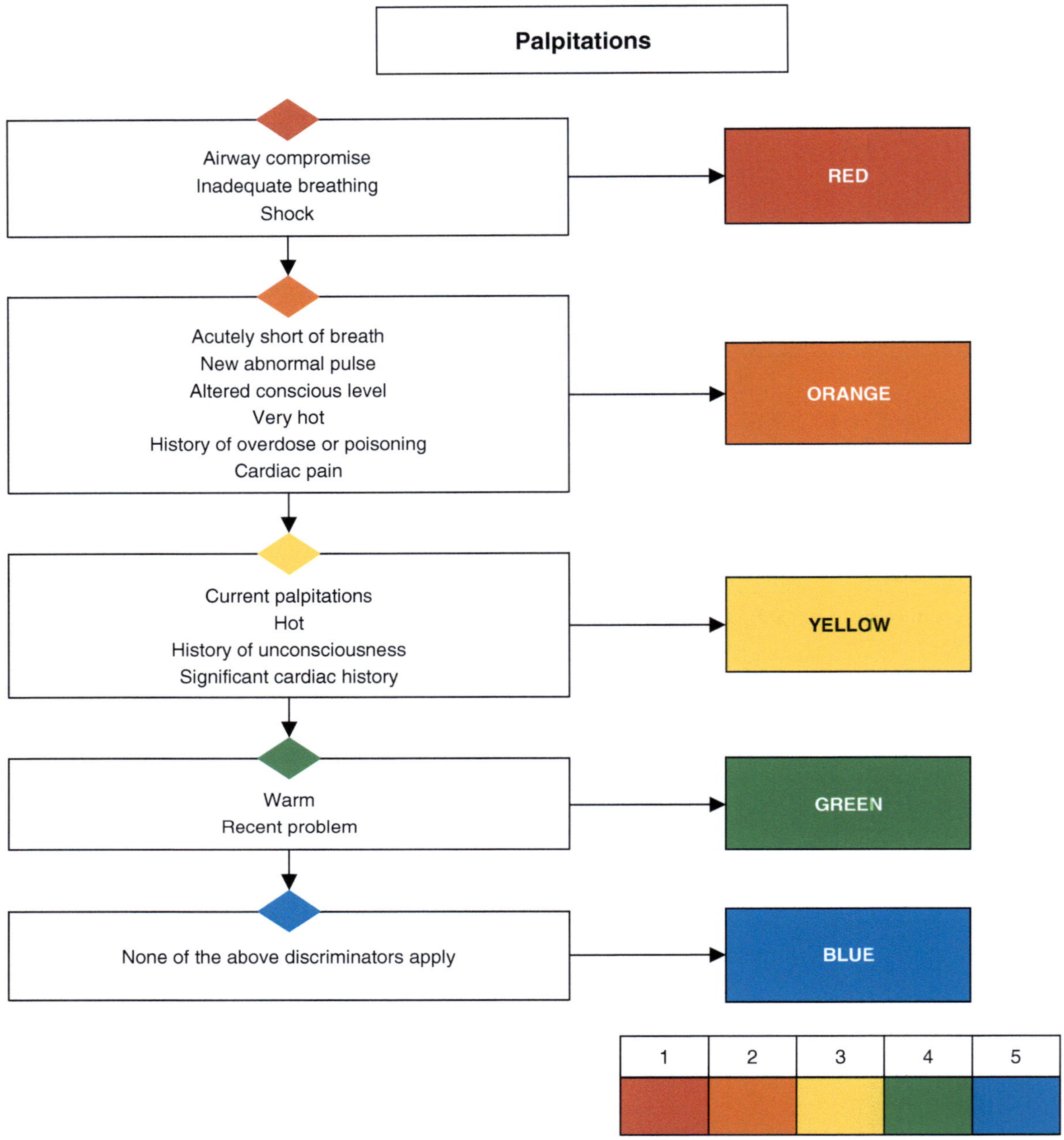
Palpitations
Airway compromise
Inadequate breathing
Shock
RED
Acutely short of breath
New abnormal pulse
Altered conscious level
Very hot
History of overdose or poisoning
Cardiac pain
ORANGE
Current palpitations
Hot
History of unconsciousness
Significant cardiac history
YELLOW
Warm
Recent problem
GREEN
None of the above discriminators apply
BLUE
1
2
3
4
5

Notes accompanying Palpitations

Related charts	Chart notes
Chest pain Collapse Unwell adult Unwell child	This chart is designed to allow the accurate prioritisation of those patients who present with a chief complaint of palpitations. Palpitations can have many causes ranging from the effects of ischaemic heart disease and other cardiac abnormalities to anxiety. Whatever the cause, it is their effect on circulation and their propensity to develop into life-threatening dysrhythmias that determine the clinical priority of the patient. Thus this chart is written to ensure that the signs and symptoms of cardiac insufficiency are included in the RED and ORANGE categories, together with historical pointers to potential early problems

Relevant discriminators	Definition
Acutely short of breath	Shortness of breath that comes on suddenly, or a sudden exacerbation of chronic shortness of breath
New abnormal pulse	A bradycardia (less than 60/min in adults), a tachycardia (more than 100/min in adults) or an irregular rhythm. Age-appropriate definitions of bradycardia and tachycardia should be used in children
History of overdose or poisoning	This information may come from others or may be deduced if medication is missing
Cardiac pain	Classically, a severe dull 'gripping' or 'heavy' pain in the centre of the chest, radiating to the left arm or to the neck. Maybe associated with sweating and nausea. Some patients may be less likely to seek medical attention and treatment quickly, despite the warning signs
Current palpitations	A feeling of the heart racing (often described as a fluttering) that is still present
Significant cardiac history	A known recurrent dysrhythmia that has life-threatening effects is significant, as is a known cardiac condition which may deteriorate rapidly

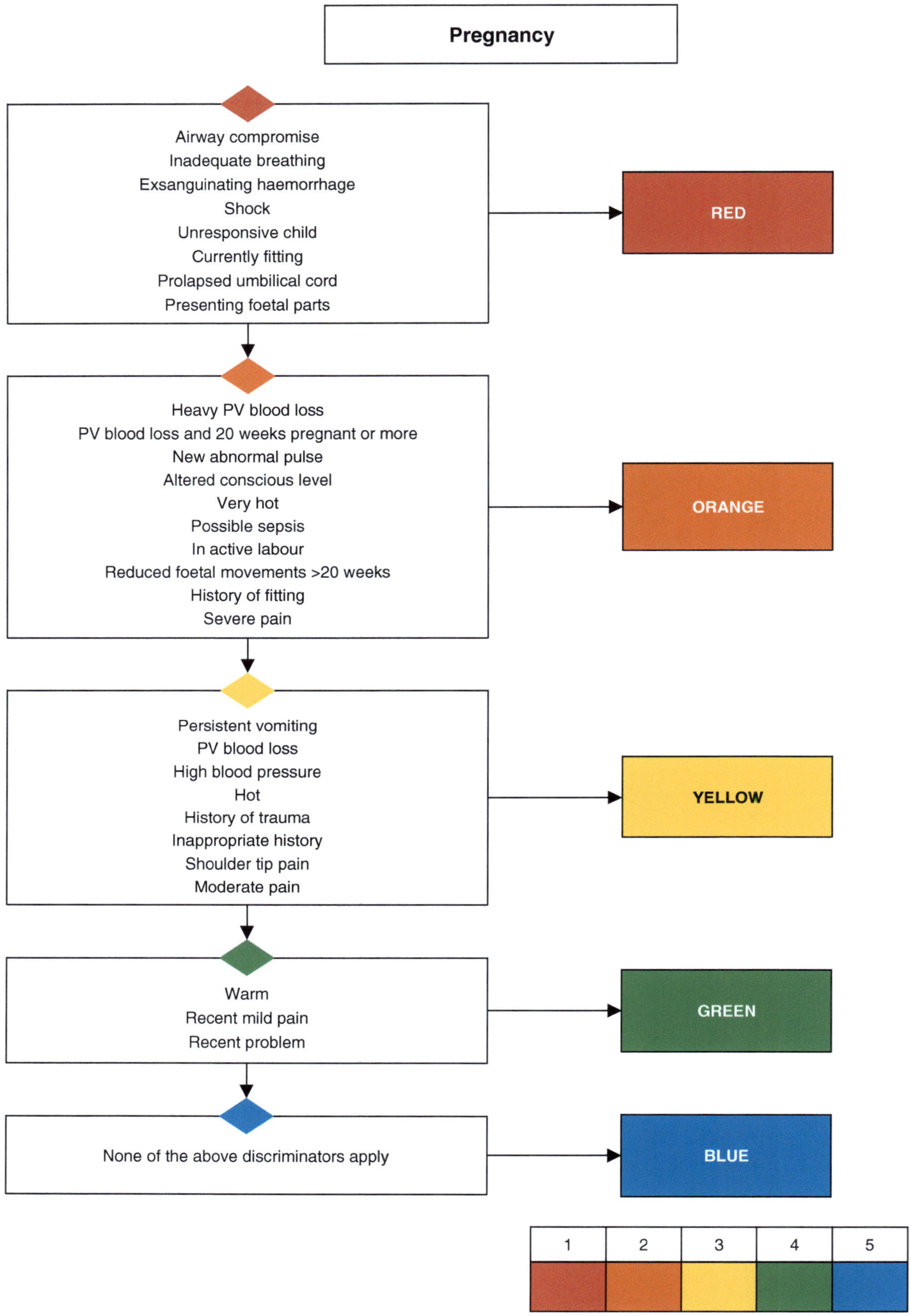
Pregnancy
Airway compromise
Inadequate breathing
Exsanguinating haemorrhage
Shock
Unresponsive child
Currently fitting
Prolapsed umbilical cord
Presenting foetal parts
RED
Heavy PV blood loss
PV blood loss and 20 weeks pregnant or more
New abnormal pulse
Altered conscious level
Very hot
Possible sepsis
In active labour
Reduced foetal movements >20 weeks
History of fitting
Severe pain
ORANGE
Persistent vomiting
PV blood loss
High blood pressure
Hot
History of trauma
Inappropriate history
Shoulder tip pain
Moderate pain
YELLOW
Warm
Recent mild pain
Recent problem
GREEN
None of the above discriminators apply
BLUE
1
2
3
4
5

Notes accompanying Pregnancy

Related charts	**Chart notes**
PV bleeding	Pregnant patients may attend urgent and emergency care at all stages of pregnancy and with a variety of complaints. Some may be unaware of their pregnancy. A number of general discriminators have been used including *Pain* and *Conscious level*. Specific discriminators are designed to allow early recognition of complications of pregnancy at all stages

Relevant discriminators	**Definition**
Prolapsed umbilical cord	Prolapse of any part of the umbilical cord through the cervix
Presenting foetal parts	Crowning or presentation of any other foetal part in the vagina
Heavy PV blood loss	PV loss is extremely difficult to assess. The presence of large clots or constant flow fulfils this criterion. The use of a large number of sanitary towels is suggestive of heavy loss
PV blood loss and 20 weeks pregnant or more	Any loss of blood PV in a patient known to be beyond the 20th week of pregnancy
In active labour	A patient who is having regular and frequent painful contractions
Reduced foetal movements >20 weeks	Absent or reduced foetal movements during the previous 12 hours in a patient known to be beyond the 20th week of pregnancy
History of fitting	Any observed or reported fits that have occurred during the period of illness or following an episode of trauma
Persistent vomiting	Vomiting that is continuous or that occurs without any respite between episodes
PV blood loss	Any loss of blood PV
High blood pressure	A history of raised blood pressure or a raised blood pressure on examination
History of trauma	A history of a recent physically traumatic event
Inappropriate history	When the history (story) given does not explain the physical findings it is termed inappropriate. This is important as it is a marker of safeguarding concerns in both adults and children
Shoulder tip pain	Pain felt in the tip of the shoulder. This often indicates diaphragmatic irritation

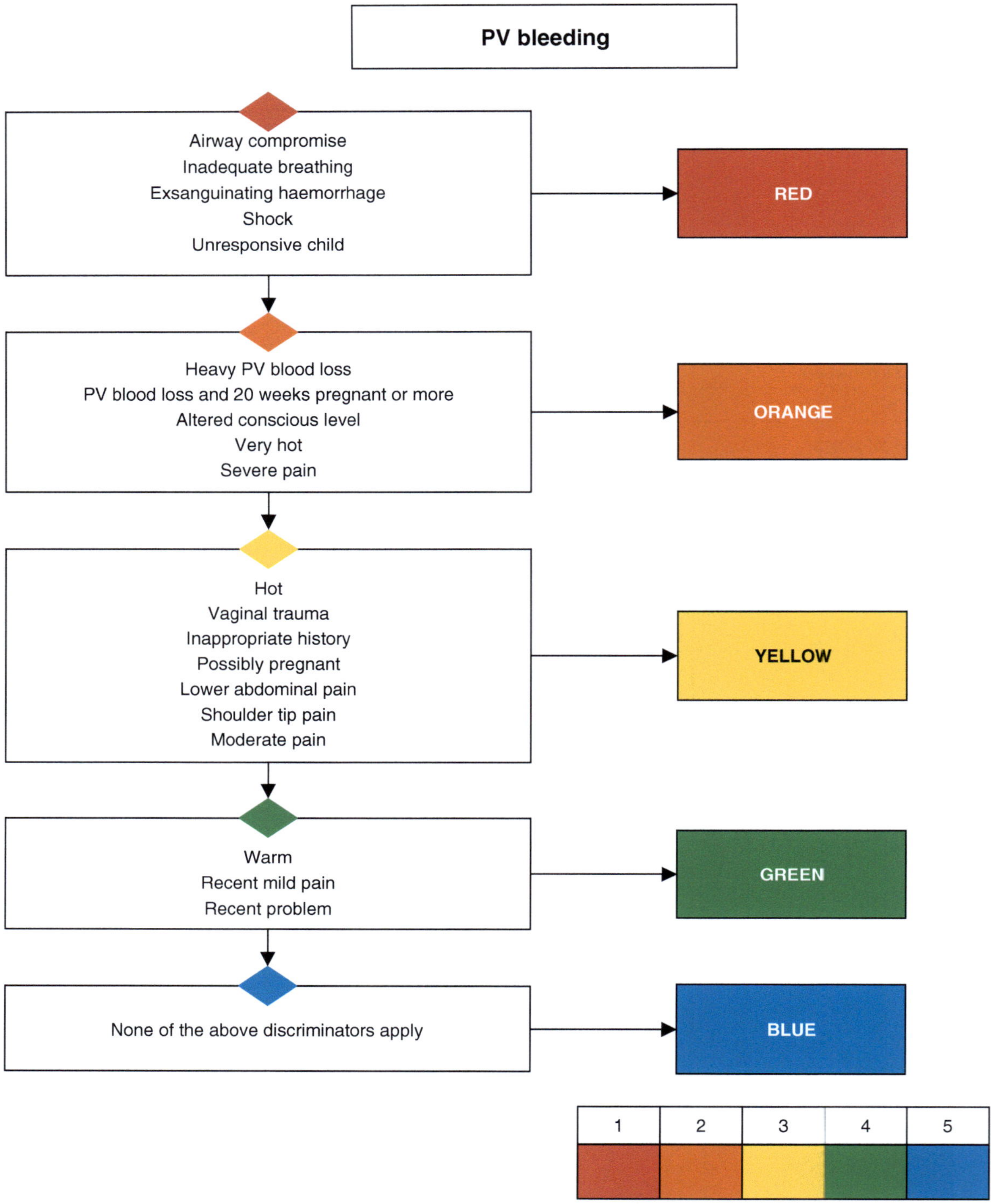
PV bleeding
Airway compromise
Inadequate breathing
Exsanguinating haemorrhage
Shock
Unresponsive child
RED
Heavy PV blood loss
PV blood loss and 20 weeks pregnant or more
Altered conscious level
Very hot
Severe pain
ORANGE
Hot
Vaginal trauma
Inappropriate history
Possibly pregnant
Lower abdominal pain
Shoulder tip pain
Moderate pain
YELLOW
Warm
Recent mild pain
Recent problem
GREEN
None of the above discriminators apply
BLUE
1
2
3
4
5

Notes accompanying PV bleeding

Related charts	Chart notes
Abdominal pain in adults Abdominal pain in children Pregnancy	PV bleeding may occur in pregnant and non-pregnant patients and may have a large number of undefined causes. A number of general discriminators are used including *Life threat*, *Haemorrhage* and *Pain*

Relevant discriminators	Definition
Heavy PV blood loss	PV loss is extremely difficult to assess. The presence of large clots or constant flow fulfils this criterion. The use of a large number of sanitary towels is suggestive of heavy loss
PV blood loss and 20 weeks pregnant or more	Any loss of blood PV in a patient known to be beyond the 20th week of pregnancy
Vaginal trauma	Any history or other evidence of direct trauma to the vagina
Inappropriate history	When the history (story) given does not explain the physical findings it is termed inappropriate. This is important as it is a marker of safeguarding concerns in both adults and children
Possibly pregnant	Any patient whose normal menstruation has failed to occur is possibly pregnant and any patient of child-bearing age who is having unprotected sex should be considered to be potentially pregnant
Lower abdominal pain	Any pain felt in the lower abdomen; in association with PV bleeding may indicate ectopic pregnancy or miscarriage
Shoulder tip pain	Pain felt in the tip of the shoulder. This often indicates diaphragmatic irritation

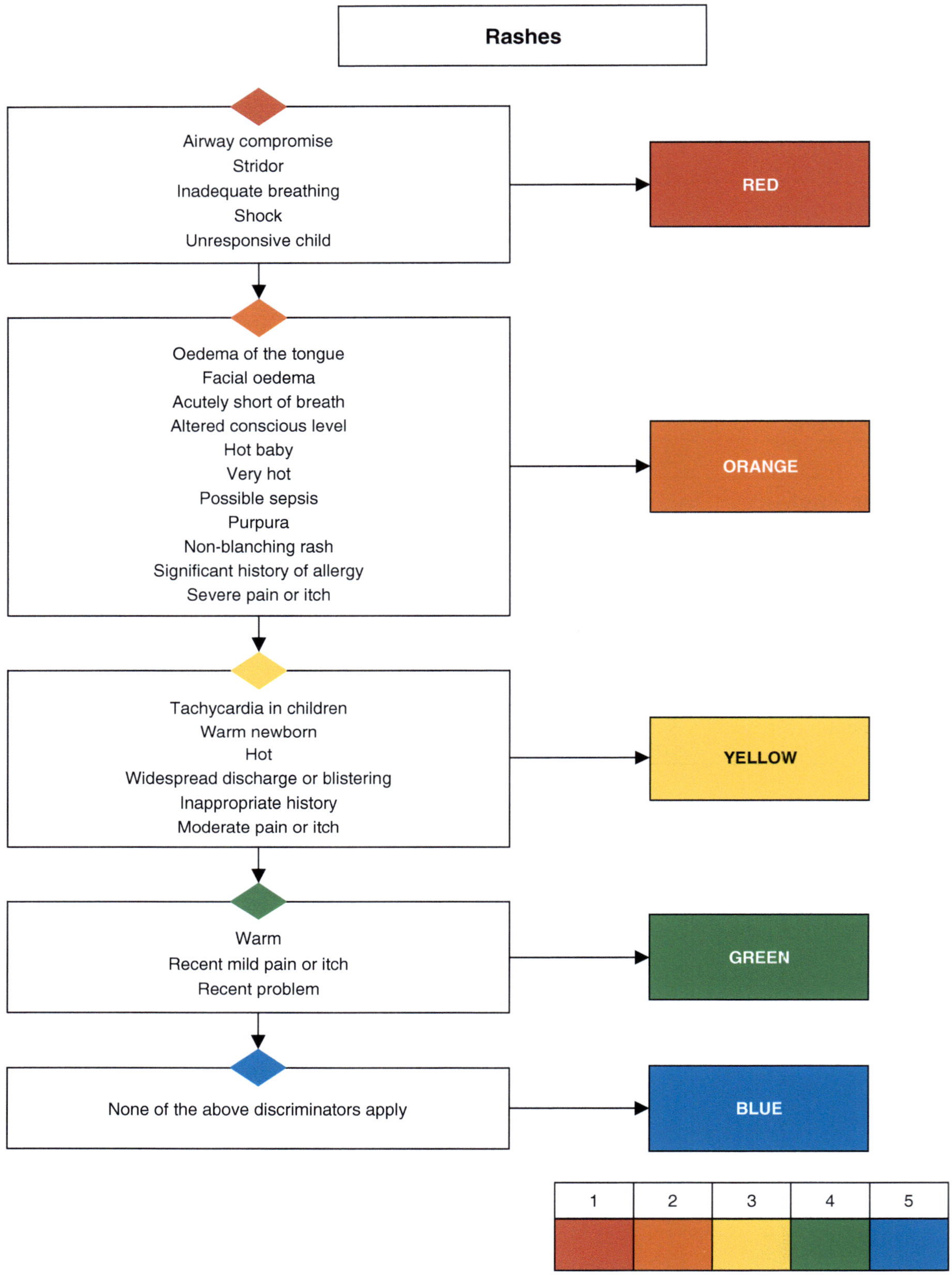
Rashes
Airway compromise
Stridor
Inadequate breathing
Shock
Unresponsive child
RED
Oedema of the tongue
Facial oedema
Acutely short of breath
Altered conscious level
Hot baby
Very hot
Possible sepsis
Purpura
Non-blanching rash
Significant history of allergy
Severe pain or itch
ORANGE
Tachycardia in children
Warm newborn
Hot
Widespread discharge or blistering
Inappropriate history
Moderate pain or itch
YELLOW
Warm
Recent mild pain or itch
Recent problem
GREEN
None of the above discriminators apply
BLUE
1
2
3
4
5

Notes accompanying Rashes

Related charts	Chart notes
Allergy Bites and stings	A rash may signify serious disease such as meningococcal septicaemia, or may be a sign of a chronic, non-acute problem such as psoriasis. Two general discriminators, *Life threat* and *Temperature*, are used in this chart. A larger number of specific discriminators are included in the ORANGE and YELLOW categories to ensure that more serious conditions are suitably triaged. In particular, purpura and associations of acute anaphylaxis appear at the ORANGE level

Relevant discriminators	Definition
Stridor	This may be an inspiratory or expiratory noise, or both. Stridor is heard best on breathing with the mouth open
Oedema of the tongue	Swelling of the tongue of any degree
Facial oedema	Diffuse swelling around the face, usually involving the lips
Acutely short of breath	Shortness of breath that comes on suddenly, or a sudden exacerbation of chronic shortness of breath
Possible sepsis	Suspected sepsis in patients who present with altered mental state, low blood pressure (systolic less than 100 mmHg) or raised respiratory rate (rate more than 22 breaths per minute) when using the qSOFA tool for assessment. Other sepsis screening tools may be used instead of qSOFA, and the relevant sepsis markers applied. In children, age-specific physiological tools should be used to determine if possibly septic
Purpura	A rash on any part of the body that is caused by small haemorrhages under the skin. A purpuric rash does not blanch (go white) when pressure is applied to it
Non-blanching rash	A rash that does not blanch (go white) when pressure is applied to it. Often tested using a glass tumbler to apply pressure as any colour change can be observed through the bottom of the tumbler
Significant history of allergy	A known sensitivity with severe reaction (e.g. to nuts or bee sting) is significant
Tachycardia in children	A child less than 1 year with a heart rate of 160 bpm or above ***OR*** a child 1 year or above with a heart rate of 140 bpm or above
Widespread discharge or blistering	Any discharging or blistering eruption covering more than 10% of the body surface area

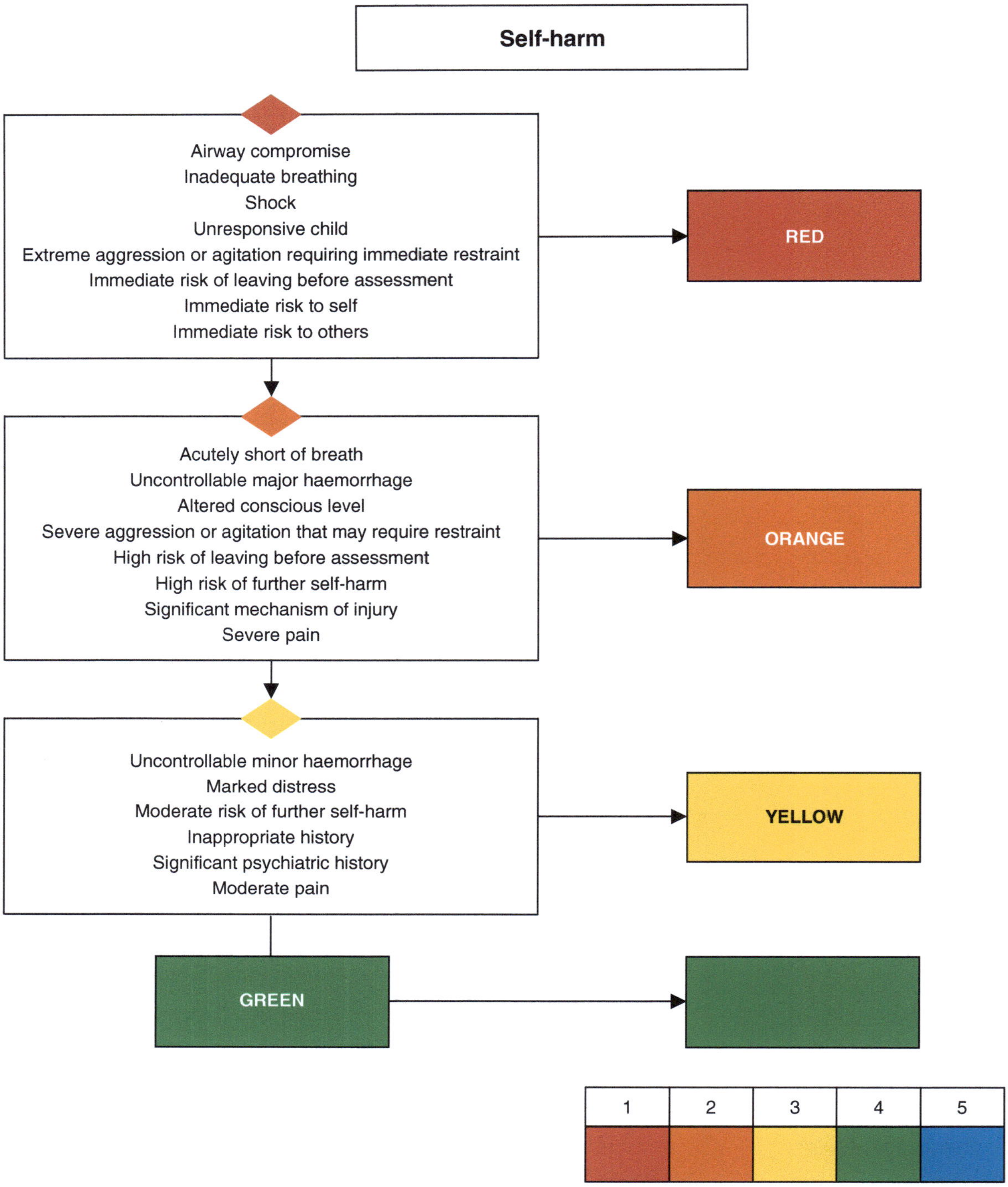
Self-harm
Airway compromise
Inadequate breathing
Shock
Unresponsive child
Extreme aggression or agitation requiring immediate restraint
Immediate risk of leaving before assessment
Immediate risk to self
Immediate risk to others
RED
Acutely short of breath
Uncontrollable major haemorrhage
Altered conscious level
Severe aggression or agitation that may require restraint
High risk of leaving before assessment
High risk of further self-harm
Significant mechanism of injury
Severe pain
ORANGE
Uncontrollable minor haemorrhage
Marked distress
Moderate risk of further self-harm
Inappropriate history
Significant psychiatric history
Moderate pain
YELLOW
GREEN
1
2
3
4
5

Notes accompanying Self-harm

Related charts	Chart notes
Mental illness Overdose and poisoning Wounds	This chart is designed to allow accurate prioritisation of patients who have caused physical harm to themselves, to allow assessment of both physical and psychiatric aspects of the presentation. A separate chart entitled Overdose and poisoning has been designed as well. A number of general discriminators are used including *Life threat*, *Haemorrhage*, *Conscious level* and *Pain*. Specific discriminators are included to allow accurate prioritisation of patients with significant mechanisms of injury and those who have various degrees of risk of further self-harm

Relevant discriminators	Definition
Extreme aggression or agitation requiring immediate restraint	Aggression and agitation of such a degree that immediate restraint is required to manage the risk of harm to self or others
Immediate risk of leaving before assessment	Active, credible attempts to leave prior to assessment pose an immediate risk
Immediate risk to self	An initial view of the risk of harm to self can be formed by considering the patient's behaviour. Patients who are actively harming themselves and those who are threatening to harm themselves and who have the means to do so are at immediate risk
Immediate risk to others	An initial view of the risk of harm to others can be judged by looking at posture (tense, clenched), speech (loud, using threatening words) and motor behaviour (restless, pacing, lunging at others). Immediate risk should be assumed if weapons and potential victims are available and no controls are already in place
Severe aggression or agitation that may require restraint	Aggression and agitation of such a degree that restraint may be required at short notice to manage the risk of harm to self or others
High risk of leaving before assessment	Active, credible threats to leave prior to assessment pose a high risk
High risk of further self-harm	An initial view of the risk of harm to self can be formed by considering the patient's behaviour. Patients who are threatening to harm themselves and who are actively seeking the means to do so are at high risk
Significant mechanism of injury	Penetrating injuries (stab or gunshot) and injuries with high energy transfer. In the frail/elderly, low energy transfer such as a fall from standing may be significant
Marked distress	Patients who are markedly physically or emotionally upset
Moderate risk of further self-harm	An initial view of the risk of harm to self can be formed by considering the patient's behaviour. Patients without a significant history of self-harm, who are not actively trying to harm themselves, but who profess the desire to harm themselves are at moderate risk
Significant psychiatric history	A history of a major psychiatric illness or event

Sexually acquired infection

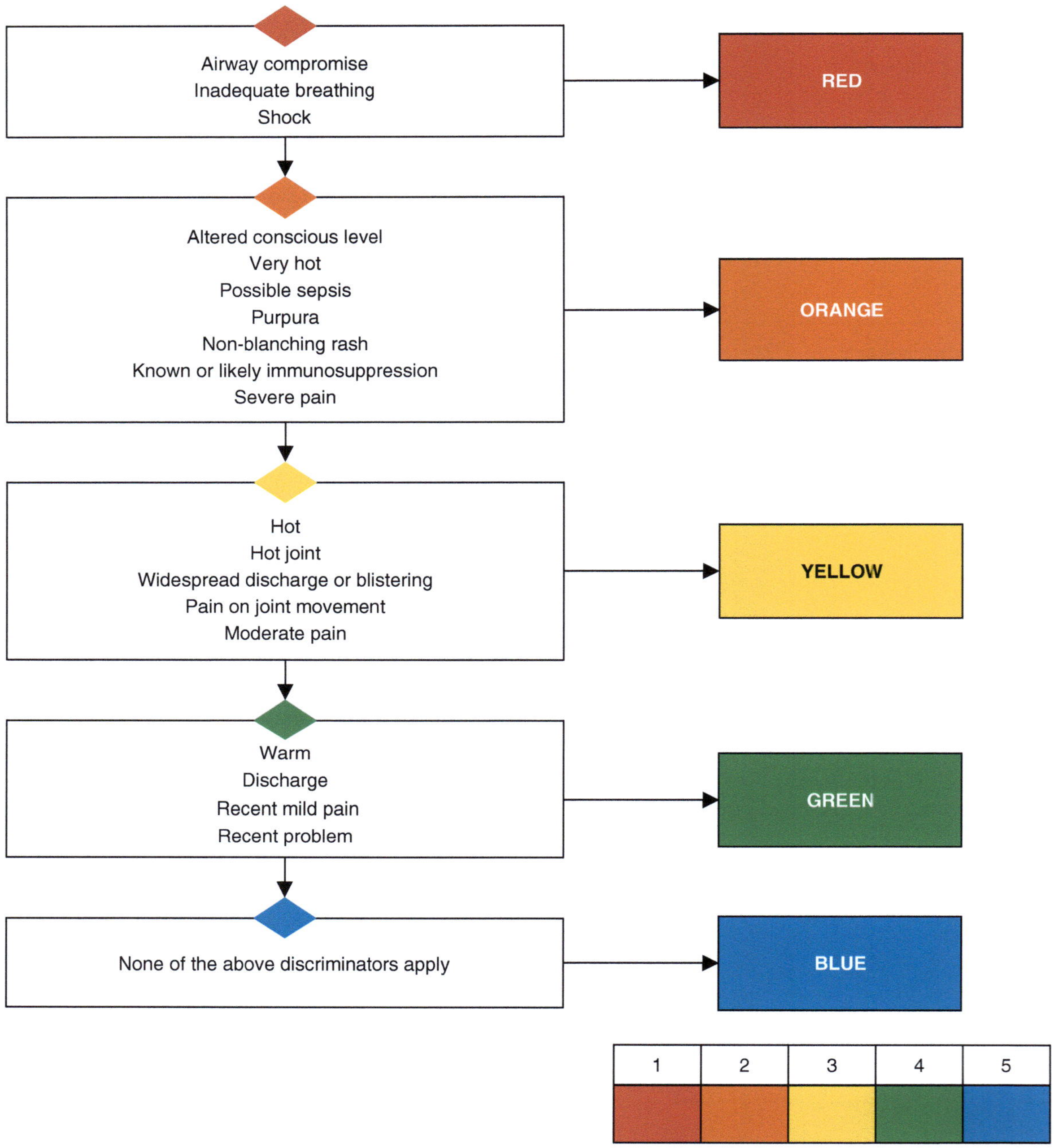

Notes accompanying Sexually acquired infection

Related charts	Chart notes
None	This chart has been included to allow prioritisation of patients who attend with known or obvious sexual acquired infection. A number of general discriminators are used including *Life threat, Pain* and *Temperature*. Specific discriminators have been added to allow identification of more urgent conditions such as gonococcaemia. It is important to ensure that preconceptions about the disposal of these patients do not prevent appropriate triage

Relevant discriminators	Definition
Purpura	A rash on any part of the body that is caused by small haemorrhages under the skin. A purpuric rash does not blanch (go white) when pressure is applied to it
Non-blanching rash	A rash that does not blanch (go white) when pressure is applied to it. Often tested using a glass tumbler to apply pressure as any colour change can be observed through the bottom of the tumbler
Known or likely immunosuppression	Any patient who is known or likely to be immunosuppressed including those on immunosuppressive drugs (including long-term steroids)
Hot joint	Any warmth around a joint. Often accompanied by redness
Widespread discharge or blistering	Any discharging or blistering eruption covering more than 10% of the body surface area
Pain on joint movement	This can be pain on either active (patient) movement or passive (examiner) movement
Discharge	In the context of sexually acquired infection this is any discharge from the penis or abnormal discharge from the vagina

Shortness of breath in adults

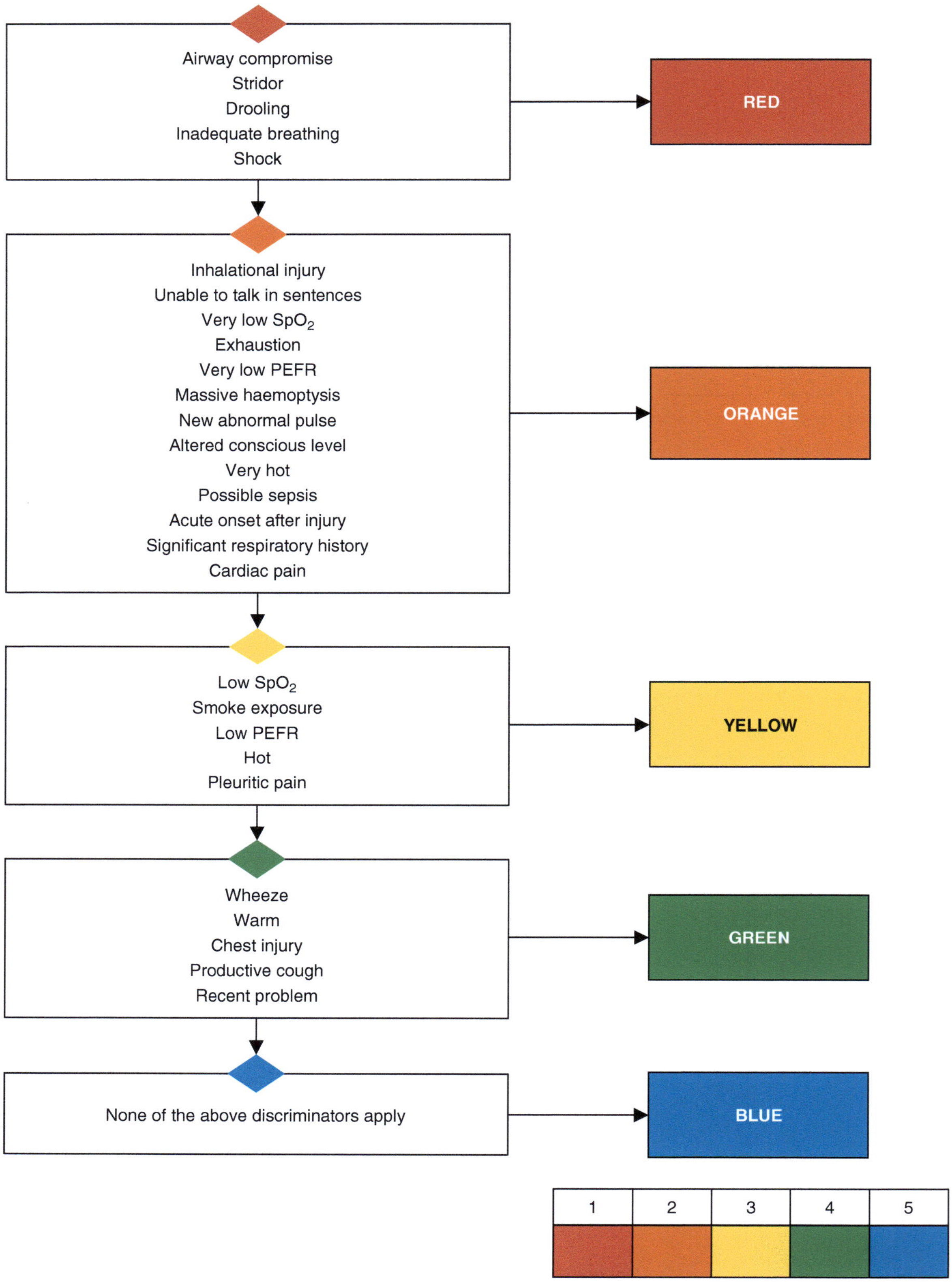

Notes accompanying Shortness of breath in adults

Related charts	Chart notes
Asthma Chest pain	Shortness of breath may be the presenting symptom for a number of cardiovascular and respiratory problems. A number of general discriminators are used including *Life threat* and *Oxygen saturation*. Specific discriminators include those which are present in severe asthma, COPD and ischaemic heart disease

Relevant discriminators	Definition
Stridor	This may be an inspiratory or expiratory noise, or both. Stridor is heard best on breathing with the mouth open
Drooling	Saliva running from the mouth as a result of being unable to swallow
Inhalational injury	A history of being confined in a smoke-filled space is the most reliable indicator of smoke inhalation. Carbon deposits around the mouth and nose and hoarse voice may be present. History is also the most reliable way of diagnosing inhalation of chemicals – there will not necessarily be any signs
Unable to talk in sentences	Patients who are so breathless that they cannot complete relatively short sentences in one breath
Very low SpO_2	This is a saturation of less than 95% on O_2 therapy or less than 92% on air. The variation in risk according to skin colour necessitates the integration of pulse oximetry with other clinical and patient-reported data
Exhaustion	Exhausted patients appear to reduce the effort they make to breathe despite continuing respiratory insufficiency. This is pre-terminal
Very low PEFR	The PEFR predicted after consideration of the age and sex of the patient. Some patients may know their 'best' PEFR and this may be used. If the ratio of measured to predicted is less than 33% then this criterion is fulfilled
Massive haemoptysis	Coughing up large amounts of fresh or clotted blood. Not to be confused with streaks of blood in saliva
Possible sepsis	Suspected sepsis in patients who present with altered mental state, low blood pressure (systolic less than 100 mmHg) or raised respiratory rate (rate more than 22 breaths per minute) when using the qSOFA tool for assessment. Other sepsis screening tools may be used instead of qSOFA, and the relevant sepsis markers applied. In children, age-specific physiological tools should be used to determine if possibly septic
Acute onset after injury	Onset of symptoms immediately within 24 hours of a physically traumatic event
Significant respiratory history	A history of previous life-threatening episodes of a respiratory condition (e.g. COPD) is significant, as is brittle asthma
Cardiac pain	Classically, a severe dull 'gripping' or 'heavy' pain in the centre of the chest, radiating to the left arm or to the neck. Maybe associated with sweating and nausea. Some patients may be less likely to seek medical attention and treatment quickly, despite the warning signs
Low SpO_2	This is a saturation of less than 95% on air. The variation in risk according to skin colour necessitates the integration of pulse oximetry with other clinical and patient-reported data
Smoke exposure	Smoke inhalation should be assumed if the patient has been confined in a smoke-filled space. Physical signs such as oral or nasal soot are less reliable but significant if present
Low PEFR	The PEFR predicted after consideration of the age and sex of the patient. Some patients may know their 'best' PEFR and this may be used. If the ratio of measured to predicted is less than 50% then this criterion is fulfilled
Pleuritic pain	A sharp, localised pain in the chest that worsens on breathing, coughing or sneezing
Wheeze	This can be audible wheeze or a feeling of wheeze. Very severe airway obstruction is silent (no air can move)
Chest injury	Any injury to the area below the clavicles and above the level of the lowest rib. Injury to the lower part of the chest can cause underlying damage to abdominal organs
Productive cough	A cough that is productive of phlegm, whatever the colour

Shortness of breath in children

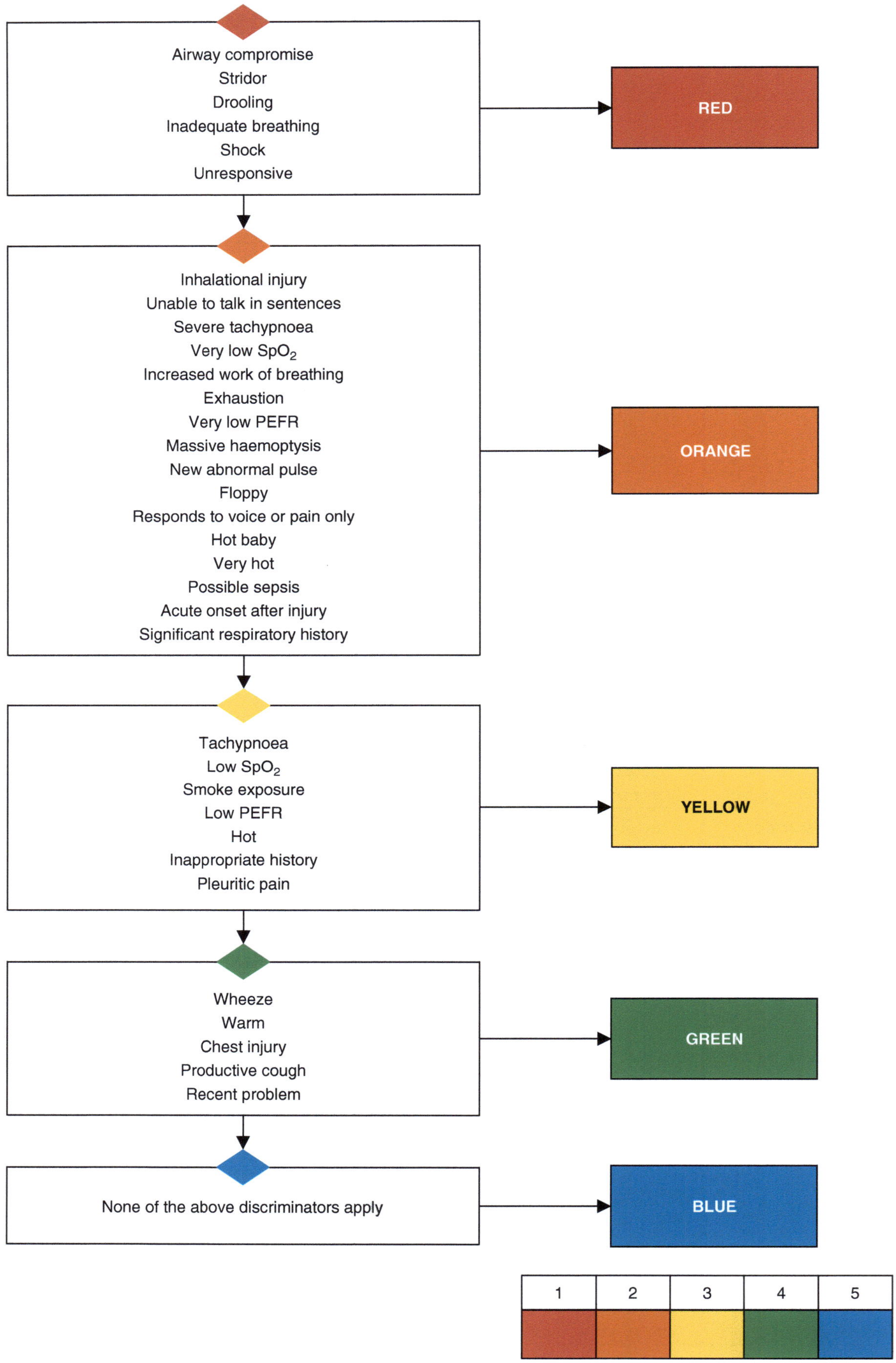

Notes accompanying Shortness of breath in children

Related charts	Chart notes
Asthma	This chart applies to children. A number of general discriminators are used including *Life threat* and *Oxygen saturation*. Specific discriminators have been included to allow accurate identification of children who are suffering the severe effects of asthma and those in whom there is more serious pathology. Accurate peak flow reading is difficult in young children and in such cases this discriminator should be ignored. Peak flow readings when obtained should always be related to the expected peak flow for age and sex

Relevant discriminators	Definition
Stridor	This may be an inspiratory or expiratory noise, or both. Stridor is heard best on breathing with the mouth open
Drooling	Saliva running from the mouth as a result of being unable to swallow
Inhalational injury	A history of being confined in a smoke-filled space is the most reliable indicator of smoke inhalation. Carbon deposits around the mouth and nose and hoarse voice may be present. History is also the most reliable way of diagnosing inhalation of chemicals – there will not necessarily be any signs
Unable to talk in sentences	Patients who are so breathless that they cannot complete relatively short sentences in one breath
Severe tachypnoea	A child less than 1 year with a respiratory rate of 55 breaths per minute or above ***OR*** a child 1 year or above with a respiratory rate of 45 breaths per minute or above
Very low SpO_2	This is a saturation of less than 95% on O_2 therapy or less than 92% on air. The variation in risk according to skin colour necessitates the integration of pulse oximetry with other clinical and patient-reported data
Increased work of breathing	Increased work of breathing is shown as increased respiratory rate, use of accessory muscles and grunting
Exhaustion	Exhausted patients appear to reduce the effort they make to breathe despite continuing respiratory insufficiency. This is pre-terminal
Very low PEFR	The PEFR predicted after consideration of the age and sex of the patient. Some patients may know their 'best' PEFR and this may be used. If the ratio of measured to predicted is less than 33% then this criterion is fulfilled
Massive haemoptysis	Coughing up large amounts of fresh or clotted blood. Not to be confused with streaks of blood in saliva
Floppy	Parents may describe their children as floppy. Tone is generally reduced – the most noticeable sign is often lolling of the head
Possible sepsis	Suspected sepsis in patients who present with altered mental state, low blood pressure (systolic less than 100 mmHg) or raised respiratory rate (rate more than 22 breaths per minute) when using the qSOFA tool for assessment. Other sepsis screening tools may be used instead of qSOFA, and the relevant sepsis markers applied. In children, age-specific physiological tools should be used to determine if possibly septic

Relevant discriminators	Definition
Acute onset after injury	Onset of symptoms immediately within 24 hours of a physically traumatic event
Significant respiratory history	A history of previous life-threatening episodes of a respiratory condition (e.g. COPD) is significant, as is brittle asthma
Tachypnoea	A child less than 1 year with a respiratory rate of 45 breaths per minute or above ***OR*** a child 1 year or above with a respiratory rate of 35 breaths per minute or above
Low SpO_2	This is a saturation of less than 95% on air. The variation in risk according to skin colour necessitates the integration of pulse oximetry with other clinical and patient-reported data
Smoke exposure	Smoke inhalation should be assumed if the patient has been confined in a smoke-filled space. Physical signs such as oral or nasal soot are less reliable but significant if present
Low PEFR	The PEFR predicted after consideration of the age and sex of the patient. Some patients may know their 'best' PEFR and this may be used. If the ratio of measured to predicted is less than 50% then this criterion is fulfilled
Inappropriate history	When the history (story) given does not explain the physical findings it is termed inappropriate. This is important as it is a marker of safeguarding concerns in both adults and children
Pleuritic pain	A sharp, localised pain in the chest that worsens on breathing, coughing or sneezing
Wheeze	This can be audible wheeze or a feeling of wheeze. Very severe airway obstruction is silent (no air can move)
Chest injury	Any injury to the area below the clavicles and above the level of the lowest rib. Injury to the lower part of the chest can cause underlying damage to abdominal organs
Productive cough	A cough that is productive of phlegm, whatever the colour

Sore throat

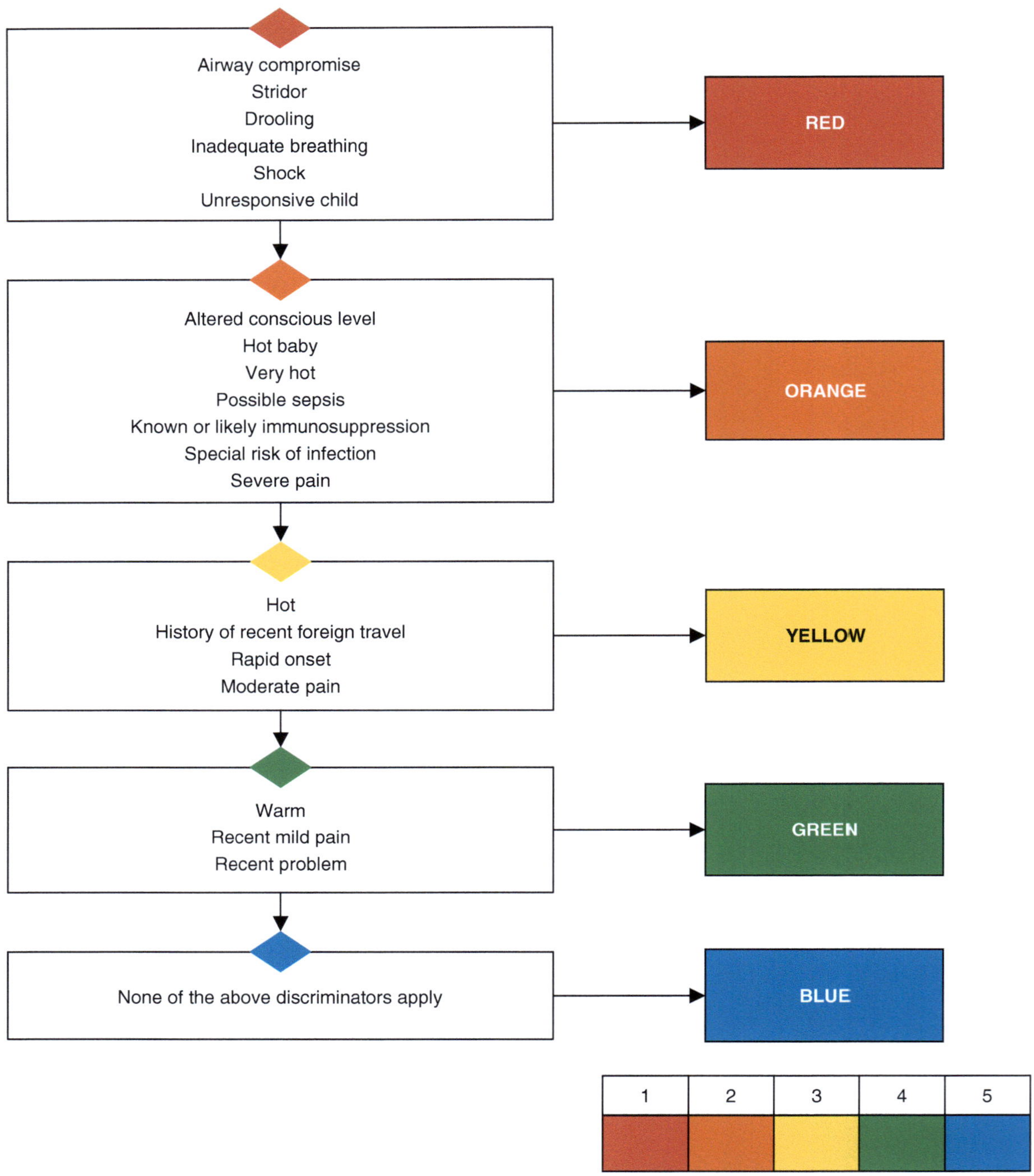
Airway compromise
Stridor
Drooling
Inadequate breathing
Shock
Unresponsive child
RED
Altered conscious level
Hot baby
Very hot
Possible sepsis
Known or likely immunosuppression
Special risk of infection
Severe pain
ORANGE
Hot
History of recent foreign travel
Rapid onset
Moderate pain
YELLOW
Warm
Recent mild pain
Recent problem
GREEN
None of the above discriminators apply
BLUE
1
2
3
4
5

Notes accompanying Sore throat

Related charts	Chart notes
Shortness of breath in adults Shortness of breath in children Unwell newborn	This chart is designed to allow accurate prioritisation for patients attending with sore throat. As problems with the throat can affect the airway there are a number of conditions that have this presentation and have a high priority. A number of general discriminators are used including *Life threat*, *Pain* and *Temperature*. Specific discriminators have been included to indicate where there is a high chance of more serious pathology. If the patient is under 28 days, the Unwell newborn chart should be used

Relevant discriminators	Definition
Stridor	This may be an inspiratory or expiratory noise, or both. Stridor is heard best on breathing with the mouth open
Drooling	Saliva running from the mouth as a result of being unable to swallow
Possible sepsis	Suspected sepsis in patients who present with altered mental state, low blood pressure (systolic less than 100 mmHg) or raised respiratory rate (rate more than 22 breaths per minute) when using the qSOFA tool for assessment. Other sepsis screening tools may be used instead of qSOFA, and the relevant sepsis markers applied. In children, age-specific physiological tools should be used to determine if possibly septic
Known or likely immunosuppression	Any patient who is known or likely to be immunosuppressed including those on immunosuppressive drugs (including long-term steroids)
Special risk of infection	Known exposure to a dangerous pathogen, or travel to an area with an identified, current, serious infectious risk
History of recent foreign travel	Recent significant foreign travel (within 2 weeks)

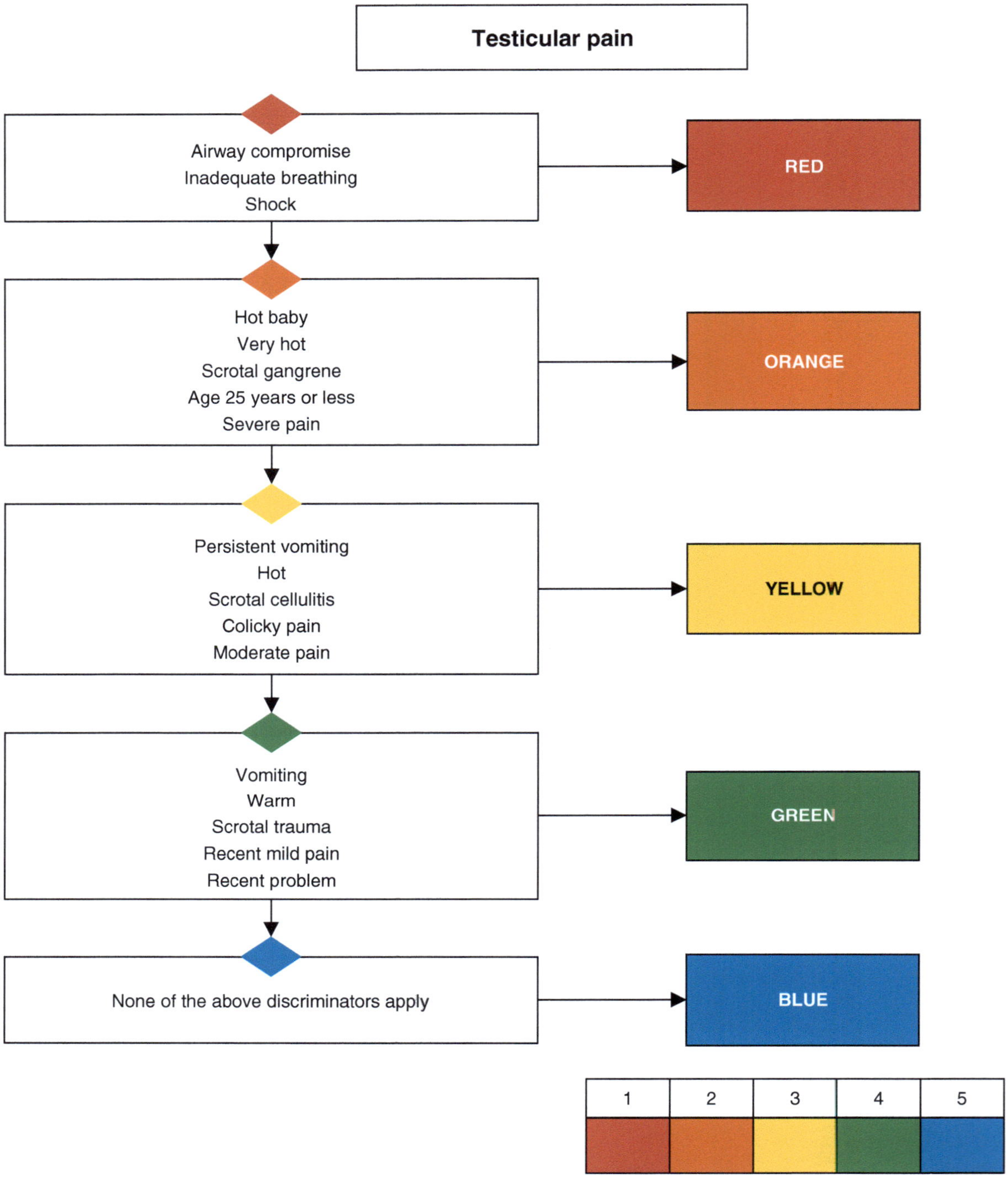
Testicular pain
Airway compromise
Inadequate breathing
Shock
RED
Hot baby
Very hot
Scrotal gangrene
Age 25 years or less
Severe pain
ORANGE
Persistent vomiting
Hot
Scrotal cellulitis
Colicky pain
Moderate pain
YELLOW
Vomiting
Warm
Scrotal trauma
Recent mild pain
Recent problem
GREEN
None of the above discriminators apply
BLUE
1
2
3
4
5

Notes accompanying Testicular pain

Related charts	Chart notes
Abdominal pain in adults Abdominal pain in children Unwell newborn	Testicular pain may have a number of pathologies, the most urgent of which is testicular torsion. A number of general discriminators are used including *Life threat*, *Pain* and *Temperature*. Specific discriminators included in the ORANGE category are designed to indicate those patients who have a high chance of torsion of the testes and the most severe infections. If the patient is under 28 days, the Unwell newborn chart should be used

Relevant discriminators	Definition
Scrotal gangrene	Dead, blackened skin around the scrotum and groin. Early gangrene may not be black but may appear like a full-thickness burn with or without flaking
Age 25 years or less	Less than 25 years old
Persistent vomiting	Vomiting that is continuous or that occurs without any respite between episodes
Scrotal cellulitis	Redness and swelling around the scrotum
Colicky pain	Pain that comes and goes in waves. Renal colic tends to come and go over 20 minutes or so
Vomiting	Any emesis
Scrotal trauma	Any recent physically traumatic event involving the scrotum

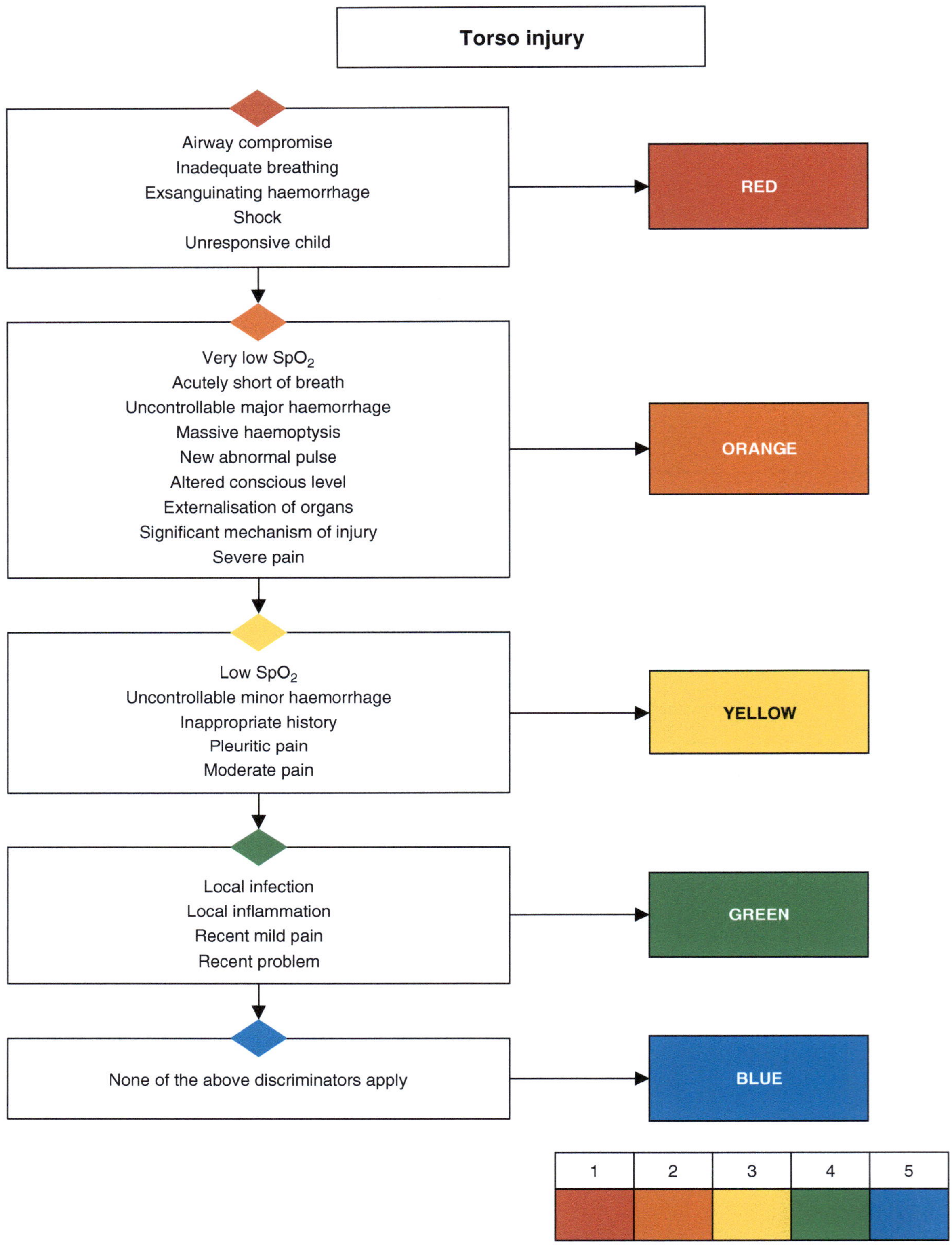
Torso injury
Airway compromise
Inadequate breathing
Exsanguinating haemorrhage
Shock
Unresponsive child
RED
Very low SpO_2
Acutely short of breath
Uncontrollable major haemorrhage
Massive haemoptysis
New abnormal pulse
Altered conscious level
Externalisation of organs
Significant mechanism of injury
Severe pain
ORANGE
Low SpO_2
Uncontrollable minor haemorrhage
Inappropriate history
Pleuritic pain
Moderate pain
YELLOW
Local infection
Local inflammation
Recent mild pain
Recent problem
GREEN
None of the above discriminators apply
BLUE
1
2
3
4
5

Notes accompanying Torso injury

Related charts	Chart notes
Assault Wounds	This chart is designed to allow accurate prioritisation of patients who have suffered injuries to the front or back of the chest and abdomen. A number of general discriminators are used including *Life threat*, *Haemorrhage* and *Pain*. Specific discriminators have been used to allow the identification of patients who are suffering from less obvious but severe internal injury. These would include patients who are acutely short of breath and those with a history suggestive of significant trauma

Relevant discriminators	Definition
Very low SpO_2	This is a saturation of less than 95% on O_2 therapy or less than 92% on air. The variation in risk according to skin colour necessitates the integration of pulse oximetry with other clinical and patient-reported data
Acutely short of breath	Shortness of breath that comes on suddenly, or a sudden exacerbation of chronic shortness of breath
Massive haemoptysis	Coughing up large amounts of fresh or clotted blood. Not to be confused with streaks of blood in saliva
Externalisation of organs	Herniation or frank extrusion of internal organs
Significant mechanism of injury	Penetrating injuries (stab or gunshot) and injuries with high energy transfer. In the frail/elderly, low energy transfer such as a fall from standing may be significant
Low SpO_2	This is a saturation of less than 95% on air. The variation in risk according to skin colour necessitates the integration of pulse oximetry with other clinical and patient-reported data
Pleuritic pain	A sharp, localised pain in the chest that worsens on breathing, coughing or sneezing
Local infection	Local infection usually manifests as inflammation (pain, swelling and redness) confined to a particular site or area, with or without a collection of pus
Local inflammation	Local inflammation involves pain, swelling and redness confined to a particular site or area

Unwell adult

Airway compromise
Inadequate breathing
Shock
Currently fitting
Hypoglycaemia
→ RED

Very low SpO_2
New abnormal pulse
Altered conscious level
New neurological deficit less than 24 hours old
Very hot
Cold
Possible sepsis
Signs of meningism
Purpura
Non-blanching rash
Known or likely immunosuppression
Special risk of infection
Severe pain
→ ORANGE

Low SpO_2
New neurological deficit more than 24 hours old
Hot
Widespread discharge or blistering
History of recent foreign travel
History of unconsciousness
New confusion
Rapid onset
Significant haematological or metabolic history
Moderate pain
→ YELLOW

Warm
Recent mild pain
Recent problem
→ GREEN

None of the above discriminators apply
→ BLUE

1	2	3	4	5
Red	Orange	Yellow	Green	Blue

Notes accompanying Unwell adult

Related charts	Chart notes
Collapse	This chart is mainly made up of general discriminators and is designed to be used when a patient presents with non-specific signs and symptoms, and a more specific chart cannot be selected. A number of general discriminators are used including *Life threat*, *Conscious level*, *Pain* and *Temperature*. Specific discriminators have been included to ensure that patients with, for example, meningococcaemia are placed in the appropriate category

Relevant discriminators	Definition
Hypoglycaemia	Glucose less than 3 mmol/l
Very low SpO_2	This is a saturation of less than 95% on O_2 therapy or less than 92% on air. The variation in risk according to skin colour necessitates the integration of pulse oximetry with other clinical and patient-reported data
New neurological deficit less than 24 hours old	Any loss of neurological function that has come on within the previous 24 hours. This might include altered or lost sensation, weakness of the limbs (either transiently or permanently) and alterations in bladder or bowel function
Possible sepsis	Suspected sepsis in patients who present with altered mental state, low blood pressure (systolic less than 100 mmHg) or raised respiratory rate (rate more than 22 breaths per minute) when using the qSOFA tool for assessment. Other sepsis screening tools may be used instead of qSOFA, and the relevant sepsis markers applied. In children, age-specific physiological tools should be used to determine if possibly septic
Signs of meningism	Classically, a stiff neck together with headache and photophobia
Purpura	A rash on any part of the body that is caused by small haemorrhages under the skin. A purpuric rash does not blanch (go white) when pressure is applied to it
Non-blanching rash	A rash that does not blanch (go white) when pressure is applied to it. Often tested using a glass tumbler to apply pressure as any colour change can be observed through the bottom of the tumbler
Known or likely immunosuppression	Any patient who is known or likely to be immunosuppressed including those on immunosuppressive drugs (including long-term steroids)
Special risk of infection	Known exposure to a dangerous pathogen, or travel to an area with an identified, current, serious infectious risk
Low SpO_2	This is a saturation of less than 95% on air. The variation in risk according to skin colour necessitates the integration of pulse oximetry with other clinical and patient-reported data
New neurological deficit more than 24 hours old	Any loss of neurological function including altered or lost sensation, weakness of the limbs (either transiently or permanently) and alterations in bladder or bowel function
History of recent foreign travel	Recent significant foreign travel (within 2 weeks)
New confusion	Patients with new onset confusion
Significant haematological or metabolic history	A patient with a significant haematological condition or a congenital metabolic disorder that is known to deteriorate rapidly

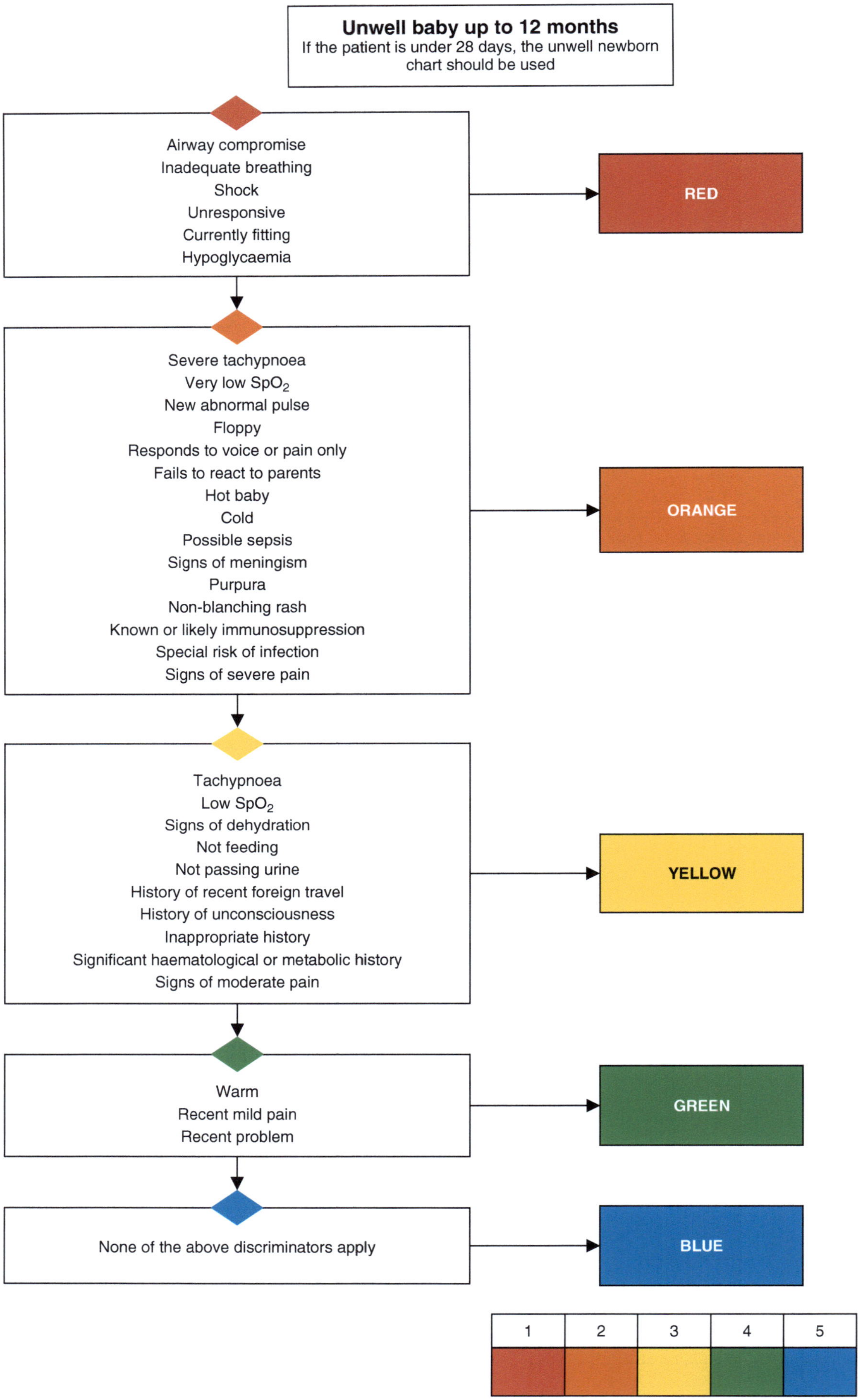
Unwell baby up to 12 months
If the patient is under 28 days, the unwell newborn chart should be used
Airway compromise
Inadequate breathing
Shock
Unresponsive
Currently fitting
Hypoglycaemia
RED
Severe tachypnoea
Very low SpO_2
New abnormal pulse
Floppy
Responds to voice or pain only
Fails to react to parents
Hot baby
Cold
Possible sepsis
Signs of meningism
Purpura
Non-blanching rash
Known or likely immunosuppression
Special risk of infection
Signs of severe pain
ORANGE
Tachypnoea
Low SpO_2
Signs of dehydration
Not feeding
Not passing urine
History of recent foreign travel
History of unconsciousness
Inappropriate history
Significant haematological or metabolic history
Signs of moderate pain
YELLOW
Warm
Recent mild pain
Recent problem
GREEN
None of the above discriminators apply
BLUE
1
2
3
4
5

Related charts	Chart notes
Crying baby Irritable child Unwell newborn Worried parent	This chart is designed to allow accurate prioritisation of babies who present with non-specific illness. A number of general discriminators are used including *Life threat*, *Conscious level*, *Pain* and *Temperature*. A number of specific discriminators have been included to allow identification of more serious pathology such as meningococcaemia, etc. If the patient is under 28 days, the Unwell newborn chart should be used

Relevant discriminators	Definition
Hypoglycaemia	Glucose less than 3 mmol/l
Severe tachypnoea	A child less than 1 year with a respiratory rate of 55 breaths per minute or above ***OR*** a child 1 year or above with a respiratory rate of 45 breaths per minute or above
Very low SpO_2	This is a saturation of less than 95% on O_2 therapy or less than 92% on air. The variation in risk according to skin colour necessitates the integration of pulse oximetry with other clinical and patient-reported data
Floppy	Parents may describe their children as floppy. Tone is generally reduced – the most noticeable sign is often lolling of the head
Fails to react to parents	Failure to react in any way to a parent's face or voice. Abnormal reactions and apparent lack of recognition of a parent are also worrying signs
Possible sepsis	Suspected sepsis in patients who present with altered mental state, low blood pressure (systolic less than 100 mmHg) or raised respiratory rate (rate more than 22 breaths per minute) when using the qSOFA tool for assessment. Other sepsis screening tools may be used instead of qSOFA, and the relevant sepsis markers applied. In children, age-specific physiological tools should be used to determine if possibly septic
Signs of meningism	Classically, a stiff neck together with headache and photophobia
Purpura	A rash on any part of the body that is caused by small haemorrhages under the skin. A purpuric rash does not blanch (go white) when pressure is applied to it
Non-blanching rash	A rash that does not blanch (go white) when pressure is applied to it. Often tested using a glass tumbler to apply pressure as any colour change can be observed through the bottom of the tumbler
Known or likely immunosuppression	Any patient who is known or likely to be immunosuppressed including those on immunosuppressive drugs (including long-term steroids)
Special risk of infection	Known exposure to a dangerous pathogen, or travel to an area with an identified, current, serious infectious risk
Tachypnoea	A child less than 1 year with a respiratory rate of 45 breaths per minute or above ***OR*** a child 1 year or above with a respiratory rate of 35 breaths per minute or above
Low SpO_2	This is a saturation of less than 95% on air. The variation in risk according to skin colour necessitates the integration of pulse oximetry with other clinical and patient-reported data
Signs of dehydration	These include dry tongue, sunken eyes, decreased skin turgor and, in small babies, a sunken anterior fontanelle. Usually associated with a low urine output
Not feeding	Children who will not take any solid or liquid (as appropriate) by mouth. Children who will take the food but always vomit afterwards may also fulfil this criterion
Not passing urine	Failure to produce and pass urine. This may be difficult to judge in children (and the elderly) and reference to the number of nappies or pads used may be useful
History of recent foreign travel	Recent significant foreign travel (within 2 weeks)
Significant haematological or metabolic history	A patient with a significant haematological condition or a congenital metabolic disorder that is known to deteriorate rapidly

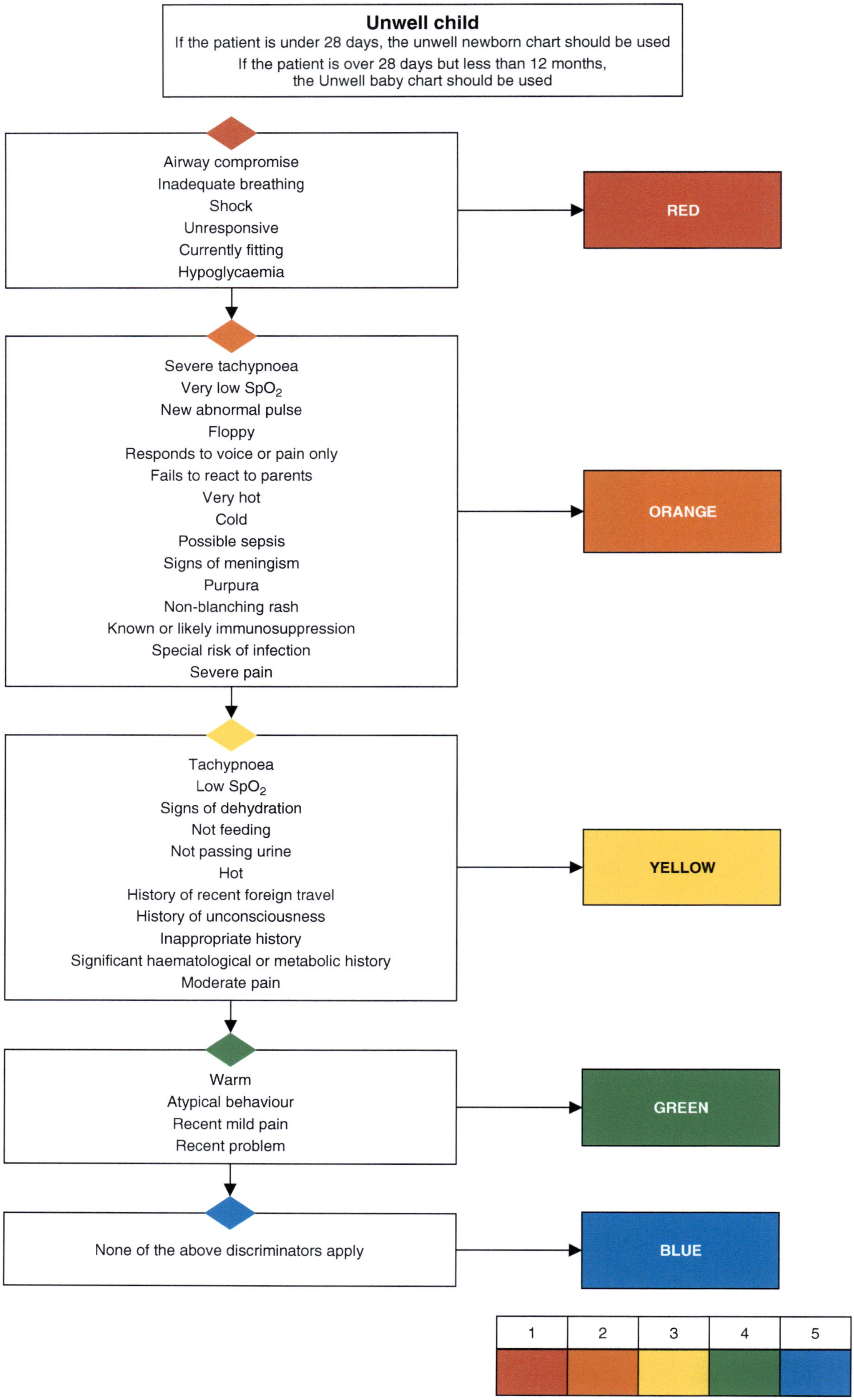
Unwell child
If the patient is under 28 days, the unwell newborn chart should be used
If the patient is over 28 days but less than 12 months, the Unwell baby chart should be used
Airway compromise
Inadequate breathing
Shock
Unresponsive
Currently fitting
Hypoglycaemia
RED
Severe tachypnoea
Very low SpO_2
New abnormal pulse
Floppy
Responds to voice or pain only
Fails to react to parents
Very hot
Cold
Possible sepsis
Signs of meningism
Purpura
Non-blanching rash
Known or likely immunosuppression
Special risk of infection
Severe pain
ORANGE
Tachypnoea
Low SpO_2
Signs of dehydration
Not feeding
Not passing urine
Hot
History of recent foreign travel
History of unconsciousness
Inappropriate history
Significant haematological or metabolic history
Moderate pain
YELLOW
Warm
Atypical behaviour
Recent mild pain
Recent problem
GREEN
None of the above discriminators apply
BLUE
1
2
3
4
5

Notes accompanying Unwell child

Related charts	Chart notes
Crying baby Irritable child Unwell newborn Worried parent	This chart is mainly made up of general discriminators and is designed to allow accurate prioritisation of children over the age of 12 months who present with non-specific signs and symptoms, and where a more specific chart cannot be chosen. A number of general discriminators are used including *Life threat*, *Conscious level*, *Pain* and *Temperature*. A number of specific discriminators have been included to allow identification of more serious pathology such as meningococcaemia, etc. If the patient is under 28 days, the Unwell newborn chart should be used

Relevant discriminators	Definition
Hypoglycaemia	Glucose less than 3 mmol/l
Severe tachypnoea	A child less than 1 year with a respiratory rate of 55 breaths per minute or above ***OR*** a child 1 year or above with a respiratory rate of 45 breaths per minute or above
Very low SpO_2	This is a saturation of less than 95% on O_2 therapy or less than 92% on air. The variation in risk according to skin colour necessitates the integration of pulse oximetry with other clinical and patient-reported data
Floppy	Parents may describe their children as floppy. Tone is generally reduced – the most noticeable sign is often lolling of the head
Fails to react to parents	Failure to react in any way to a parent's face or voice. Abnormal reactions and apparent lack of recognition of a parent are also worrying signs
Possible sepsis	Suspected sepsis in patients who present with altered mental state, low blood pressure (systolic less than 100 mmHg) or raised respiratory rate (rate more than 22 breaths per minute) when using the qSOFA tool for assessment. Other sepsis screening tools may be used instead of qSOFA, and the relevant sepsis markers applied. In children, age-specific physiological tools should be used to determine if possibly septic
Signs of meningism	Classically, a stiff neck together with headache and photophobia
Purpura	A rash on any part of the body that is caused by small haemorrhages under the skin. A purpuric rash does not blanch (go white) when pressure is applied to it
Non-blanching rash	A rash that does not blanch (go white) when pressure is applied to it. Often tested using a glass tumbler to apply pressure as any colour change can be observed through the bottom of the tumbler
Known or likely immunosuppression	Any patient who is known or likely to be immunosuppressed including those on immunosuppressive drugs (including long-term steroids)
Special risk of infection	Known exposure to a dangerous pathogen, or travel to an area with an identified, current, serious infectious risk
Tachypnoea	A child less than 1 year with a respiratory rate of 45 breaths per minute or above ***OR*** a child 1 year or above with a respiratory rate of 35 breaths per minute or above
Low SpO_2	This is a saturation of less than 95% on air. The variation in risk according to skin colour necessitates the integration of pulse oximetry with other clinical and patient-reported data
Signs of dehydration	These include dry tongue, sunken eyes, decreased skin turgor and, in small babies, a sunken anterior fontanelle. Usually associated with a low urine output
Not feeding	Children who will not take any solid or liquid (as appropriate) by mouth. Children who will take the food but always vomit afterwards may also fulfil this criterion.
Not passing urine	Failure to produce and pass urine. This may be difficult to judge in children (and the elderly) and reference to the number of nappies or pads used may be useful
History of recent foreign travel	Recent significant foreign travel (within 2 weeks)
Significant haematological or metabolic history	A patient with a significant haematological condition or a congenital metabolic disorder that is known to deteriorate rapidly
Atypical behaviour	Children who are behaving in a way that is not usual in the given situation. The carers will often volunteer this information. Such children are often referred to as fractious or 'out of sorts'

Unwell newborn up to 28 days

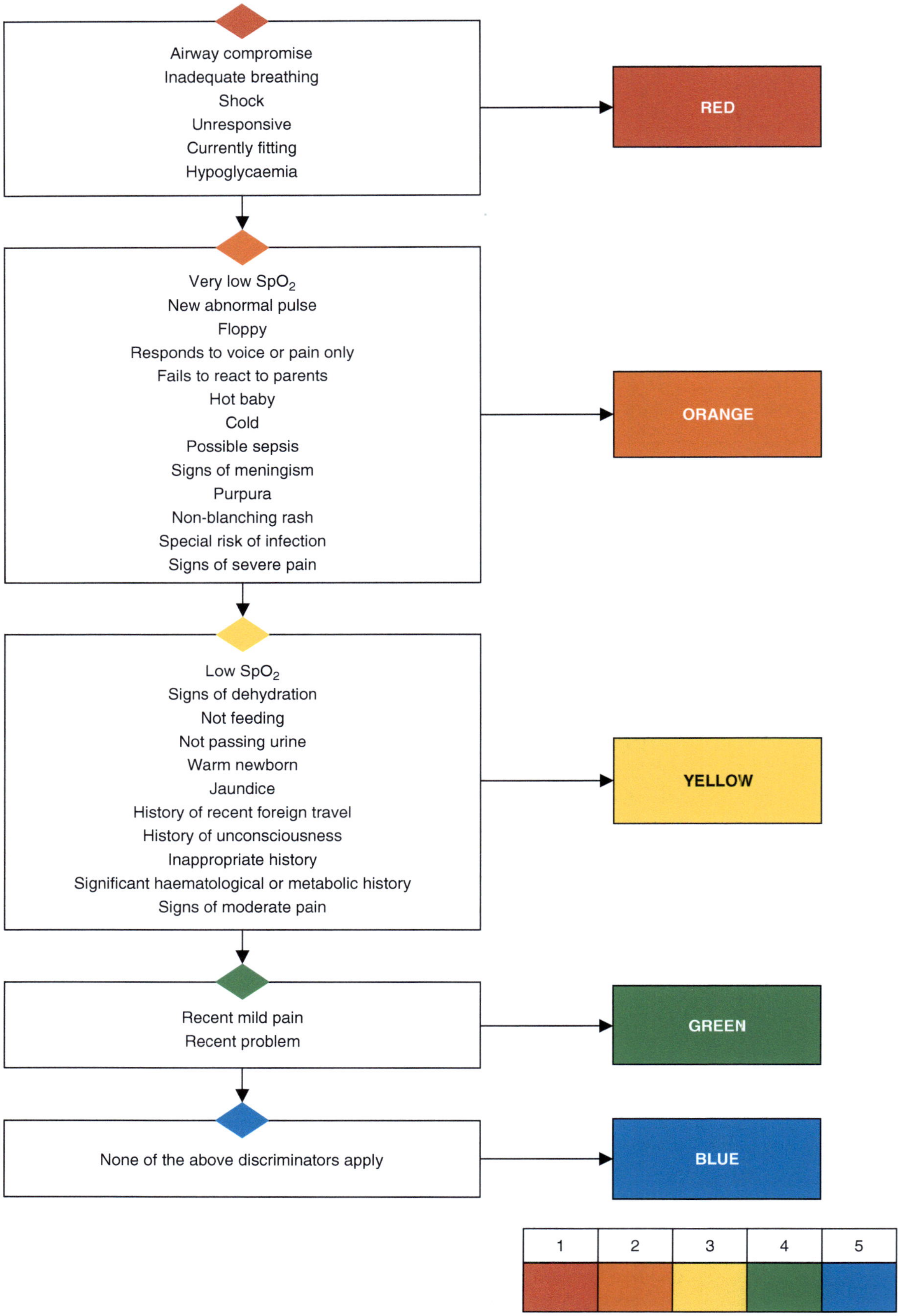

Notes accompanying Unwell newborn up to 28 days

Related charts	Chart notes
None	This chart is designed to allow accurate prioritisation of newborns (up to 28 days) who present with non-specific illness. A number of general discriminators are used including *Life threat*, *Conscious level*, *Pain* and *Temperature*. A number of specific discriminators have been included to allow identification of more serious pathology such as meningococcaemia, etc.

Relevant discriminators	Definition
Hypoglycaemia	Glucose less than 3 mmol/l
Very low SpO_2	This is a saturation of less than 95% on O_2 therapy or less than 92% on air. The variation in risk according to skin colour necessitates the integration of pulse oximetry with other clinical and patient-reported data
Floppy	Parents may describe their children as floppy. Tone is generally reduced – the most noticeable sign is often lolling of the head
Fails to react to parents	Failure to react in any way to a parent's face or voice. Abnormal reactions and apparent lack of recognition of a parent are also worrying signs
Possible sepsis	Suspected sepsis in patients who present with altered mental state, low blood pressure (systolic less than 100 mmHg) or raised respiratory rate (rate more than 22 breaths per minute) when using the qSOFA tool for assessment. Other sepsis screening tools may be used instead of qSOFA, and the relevant sepsis markers applied. In children, age-specific physiological tools should be used to determine if possibly septic
Signs of meningism	Classically, a stiff neck together with headache and photophobia
Purpura	A rash on any part of the body that is caused by small haemorrhages under the skin. A purpuric rash does not blanch (go white) when pressure is applied to it
Non-blanching rash	A rash that does not blanch (go white) when pressure is applied to it. Often tested using a glass tumbler to apply pressure as any colour change can be observed through the bottom of the tumbler
Special risk of infection	Known exposure to a dangerous pathogen, or travel to an area with an identified, current, serious infectious risk
Signs of severe pain	Young children and babies in severe pain cannot complain. They will usually cry out continuously and inconsolably and be tachycardic. They may well exhibit signs such as pallor and sweating
Low SpO_2	This is a saturation of less than 95% on air. The variation in risk according to skin colour necessitates the integration of pulse oximetry with other clinical and patient-reported data
Signs of dehydration	These include dry tongue, sunken eyes, decreased skin turgor and, in small babies, a sunken anterior fontanelle. Usually associated with a low urine output
Not feeding	Children who will not take any solid or liquid (as appropriate) by mouth. Children who will take the food but always vomit afterwards may also fulfil this criterion
Not passing urine	Failure to produce and pass urine. This may be difficult to judge in children (and the elderly) and reference to the number of nappies or pads used may be useful
Jaundice	Neonatal jaundice
History of recent foreign travel	Recent significant foreign travel (within 2 weeks)
Significant haematological or metabolic history	A patient with a significant haematological condition or a congenital metabolic disorder that is known to deteriorate rapidly

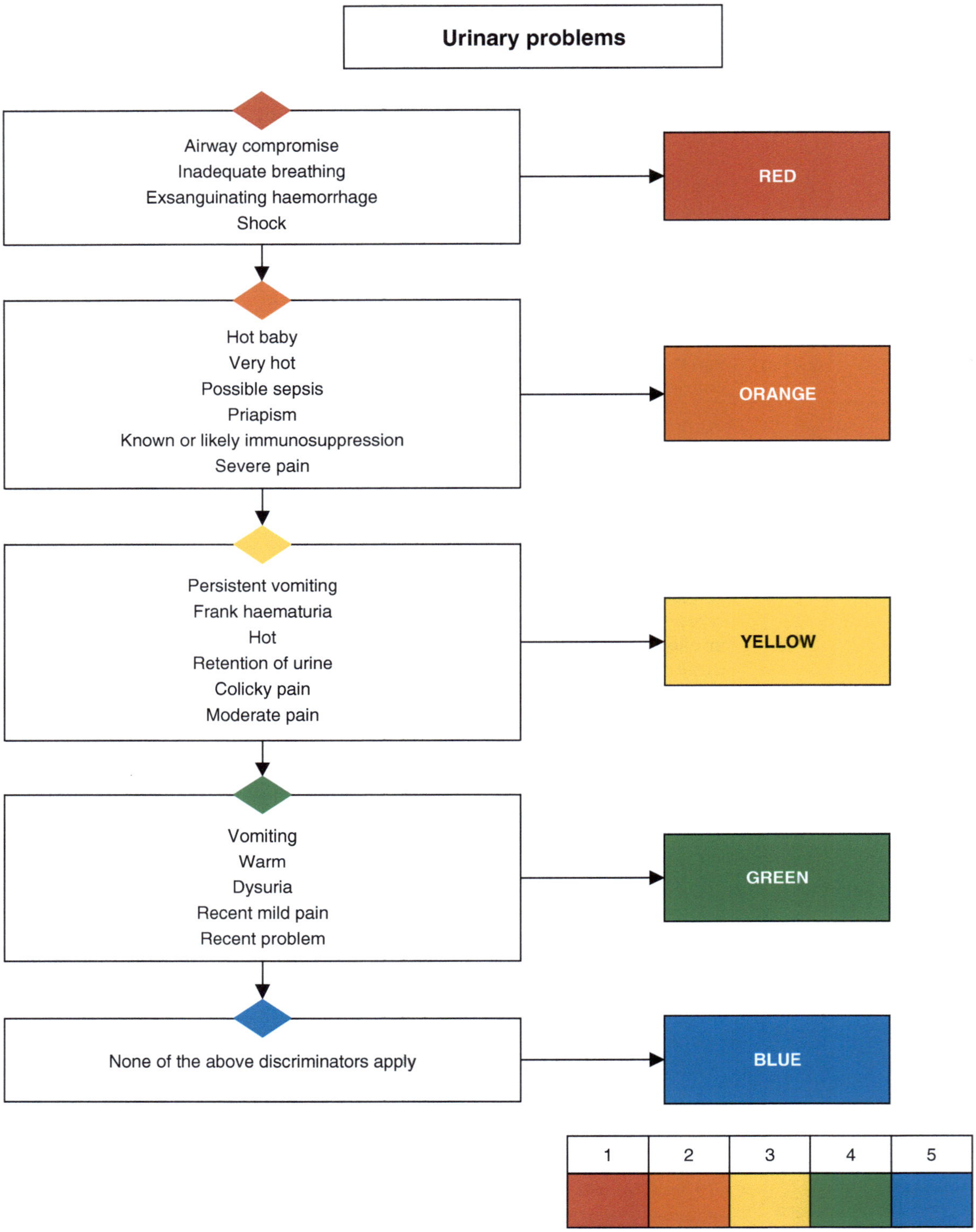
Urinary problems
Airway compromise
Inadequate breathing
Exsanguinating haemorrhage
Shock
RED
Hot baby
Very hot
Possible sepsis
Priapism
Known or likely immunosuppression
Severe pain
ORANGE
Persistent vomiting
Frank haematuria
Hot
Retention of urine
Colicky pain
Moderate pain
YELLOW
Vomiting
Warm
Dysuria
Recent mild pain
Recent problem
GREEN
None of the above discriminators apply
BLUE
1
2
3
4
5

Notes accompanying Urinary problems

Related charts	**Chart notes**
Sexually acquired infection Testicular pain Unwell newborn	Many patients who present with urinary problems are in pain and some may have serious underlying pathology. A number of general discriminators are used including *Life threat*, *Pain* and *Temperature*. Specific discriminators have been included to ensure that patients suffering from urinary retention and those with infections are included in the appropriate categories. If the patient is under 28 days, the Unwell newborn chart should be used

Relevant discriminators	**Definition**
Possible sepsis	Suspected sepsis in patients who present with altered mental state, low blood pressure (systolic less than 100 mmHg) or raised respiratory rate (rate more than 22 breaths per minute) when using the qSOFA tool for assessment. Other sepsis screening tools may be used instead of qSOFA, and the relevant sepsis markers applied. In children, age-specific physiological tools should be used to determine if possibly septic
Priapism	Sustained penile erection
Known or likely immunosuppression	Any patient who is known or likely to be immunosuppressed including those on immunosuppressive drugs (including long-term steroids)
Persistent vomiting	Vomiting that is continuous or that occurs without any respite between episodes
Frank haematuria	Red discolouration of the urine caused by blood
Retention of urine	Inability to pass urine per urethra associated with an enlarged bladder. This condition is usually very painful unless there is altered sensation
Colicky pain	Pain that comes and goes in waves. Renal colic tends to come and go over 20 minutes or so
Vomiting	Any emesis
Dysuria	Pain or difficulty in passing urine. Pain is typically described as stinging or hot

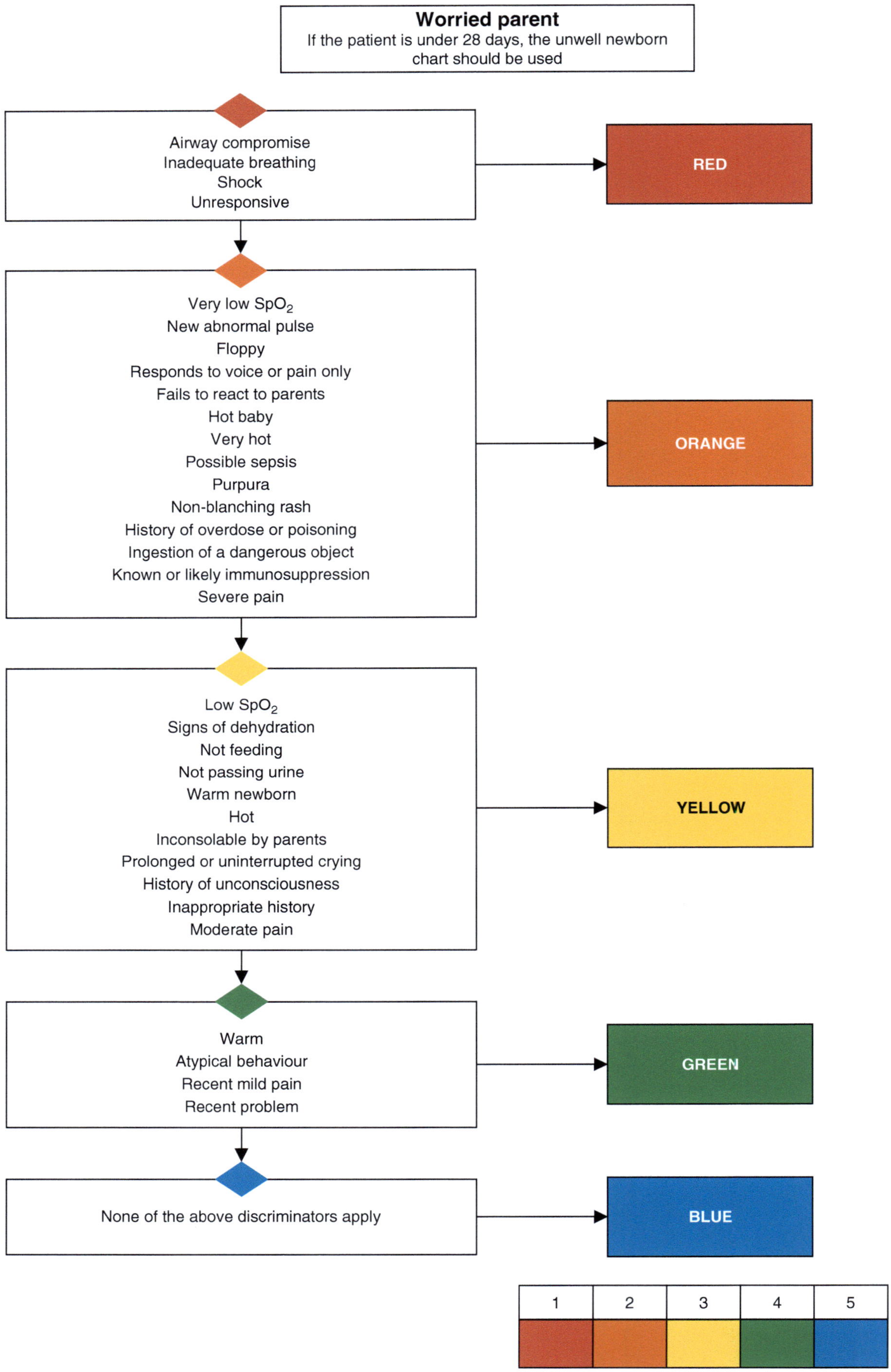
Worried parent
If the patient is under 28 days, the unwell newborn chart should be used
Airway compromise
Inadequate breathing
Shock
Unresponsive
RED
Very low SpO_2
New abnormal pulse
Floppy
Responds to voice or pain only
Fails to react to parents
Hot baby
Very hot
Possible sepsis
Purpura
Non-blanching rash
History of overdose or poisoning
Ingestion of a dangerous object
Known or likely immunosuppression
Severe pain
ORANGE
Low SpO_2
Signs of dehydration
Not feeding
Not passing urine
Warm newborn
Hot
Inconsolable by parents
Prolonged or uninterrupted crying
History of unconsciousness
Inappropriate history
Moderate pain
YELLOW
Warm
Atypical behaviour
Recent mild pain
Recent problem
GREEN
None of the above discriminators apply
BLUE
1
2
3
4
5

Notes accompanying Worried parent

Related charts	Chart notes
Crying baby Irritable child Unwell baby Unwell child Unwell newborn	This chart is designed to allow accurate prioritisation of children who are brought to the attention of the service because of parental worry. Parents know their children better than anyone else and although many of these children will not have serious pathology it is essential that these presentations are taken seriously. A number of general discriminators are used including *Life threat*, *Conscious level*, *Pain* and *Temperature*. Specific discriminators have been added to the chart to allow identification of more serious pathologies which are apparent or may potentially exist. If the patient is under 28 days, the Unwell newborn chart should be used

Relevant discriminators	Definition
Very low SpO_2	This is a saturation of less than 95% on O_2 therapy or less than 92% on air. The variation in risk according to skin colour necessitates the integration of pulse oximetry with other clinical and patient-reported data
Floppy	Parents may describe their children as floppy. Tone is generally reduced – the most noticeable sign is often lolling of the head
Fails to react to parents	Failure to react in any way to a parent's face or voice. Abnormal reactions and apparent lack of recognition of a parent are also worrying signs
Possible sepsis	Suspected sepsis in patients who present with altered mental state, low blood pressure (systolic less than 100 mmHg) or raised respiratory rate (rate more than 22 breaths per minute) when using the qSOFA tool for assessment. Other sepsis screening tools may be used instead of qSOFA, and the relevant sepsis markers applied. In children, age-specific physiological tools should be used to determine if possibly septic
Purpura	A rash on any part of the body that is caused by small haemorrhages under the skin. A purpuric rash does not blanch (go white) when pressure is applied to it
Non-blanching rash	A rash that does not blanch (go white) when pressure is applied to it. Often tested using a glass tumbler to apply pressure as any colour change can be observed through the bottom of the tumbler
History of overdose or poisoning	This information may come from others or may be deduced if medication is missing
Ingestion of a dangerous object	Ingestion of a dangerous or potentially dangerous foreign object, e.g. button battery, magnets or razor blades, which may be a potential threat to life
Known or likely immunosuppression	Any patient who is known or likely to be immunosuppressed including those on immunosuppressive drugs (including long-term steroids)
Low SpO_2	This is a saturation of less than 95% on air. The variation in risk according to skin colour necessitates the integration of pulse oximetry with other clinical and patient-reported data
Signs of dehydration	These include dry tongue, sunken eyes, decreased skin turgor and, in small babies, a sunken anterior fontanelle. Usually associated with a low urine output
Not feeding	Children who will not take any solid or liquid (as appropriate) by mouth. Children who will take the food but always vomit afterwards may also fulfil this criterion
Not passing urine	Failure to produce and pass urine. This may be difficult to judge in children (and the elderly) and reference to the number of nappies or pads used may be useful
Inconsolable by parents	Children whose crying or distress does not respond to attempts by their parents to comfort them
Prolonged or uninterrupted crying	A child who has cried continuously for 2 hours or more
Inappropriate history	When the history (story) given does not explain the physical findings it is termed inappropriate. This is important as it is a marker of safeguarding concerns in both adults and children
Atypical behaviour	Children who are behaving in a way that is not usual in the given situation. The carers will often volunteer this information. Such children are often referred to as fractious or 'out of sorts'

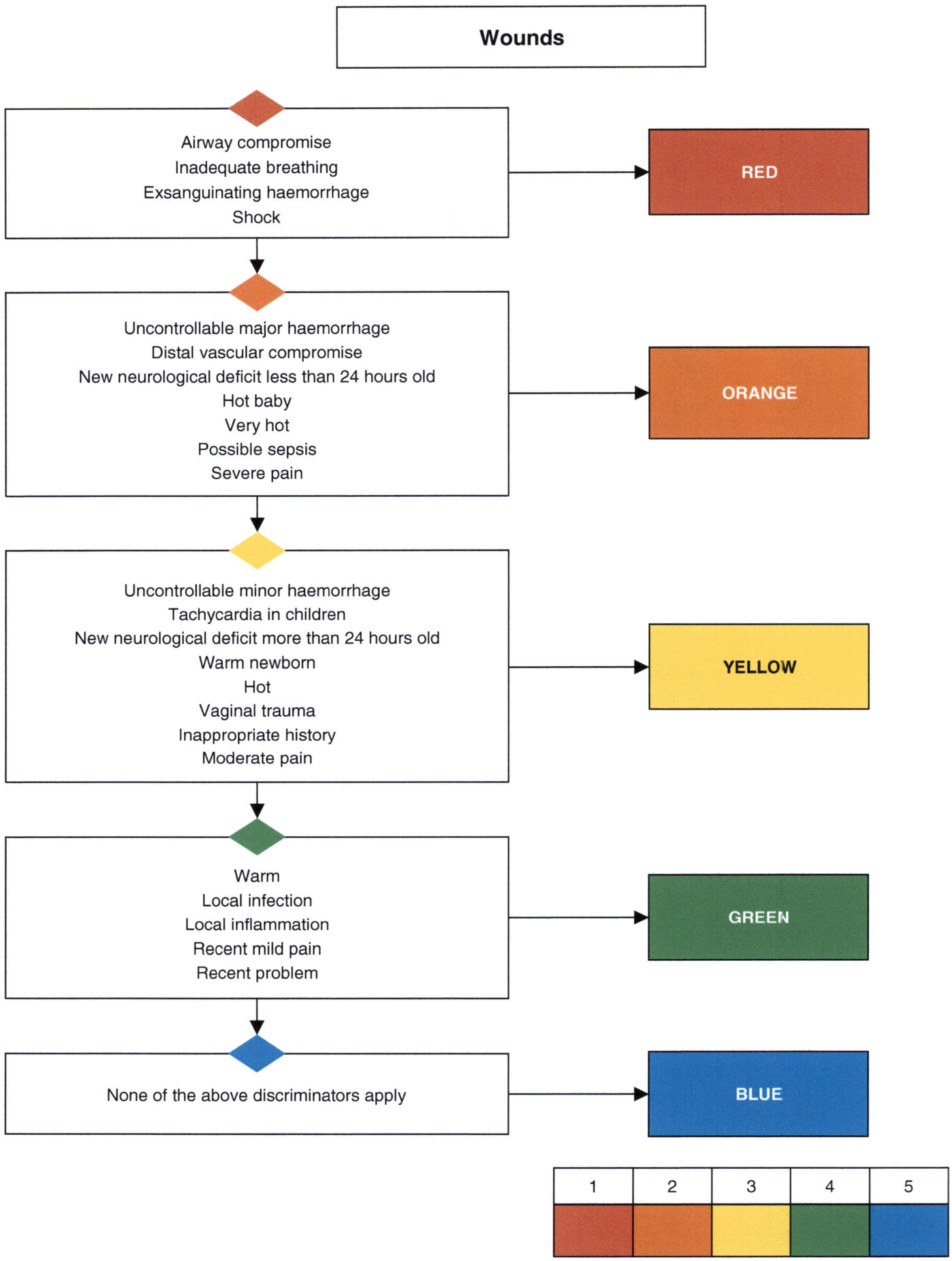
Wounds
Airway compromise
Inadequate breathing
Exsanguinating haemorrhage
Shock
RED
Uncontrollable major haemorrhage
Distal vascular compromise
New neurological deficit less than 24 hours old
Hot baby
Very hot
Possible sepsis
Severe pain
ORANGE
Uncontrollable minor haemorrhage
Tachycardia in children
New neurological deficit more than 24 hours old
Warm newborn
Hot
Vaginal trauma
Inappropriate history
Moderate pain
YELLOW
Warm
Local infection
Local inflammation
Recent mild pain
Recent problem
GREEN
None of the above discriminators apply
BLUE
1
2
3
4
5

Notes accompanying Wounds

Related charts	Chart notes
Assault	Many patients attend all forms of emergency care suffering from wounds of varying nature. These vary from severe life-threatening lacerations to minor abrasions. This chart is designed to allow an accurate prioritisation of these patients. A number of general discriminators have been used including *Life threat*, *Haemorrhage* and *Pain*. Specific discriminators have been included to allow identification of patients with signs and symptoms suggesting injuries that pose a threat to function

Relevant discriminators	Definition
Distal vascular compromise	There will be a combination of pallor, coldness, altered sensation and pain with or without absent pulses distal to the injury
New neurological deficit less than 24 hours old	Any loss of neurological function that has come on within the previous 24 hours. This might include altered or lost sensation, weakness of the limbs (either transiently or permanently) and alterations in bladder or bowel function
Possible sepsis	Suspected sepsis in patients who present with altered mental state, low blood pressure (systolic less than 100 mmHg) or raised respiratory rate (rate more than 22 breaths per minute) when using the qSOFA tool for assessment. Other sepsis screening tools may be used instead of qSOFA, and the relevant sepsis markers applied. In children, age-specific physiological tools should be used to determine if possibly septic
Tachycardia in children	A child less than 1 year with a heart rate of 160 bpm or above ***OR*** a child 1 year or above with a heart rate of 140 bpm or above
New neurological deficit more than 24 hours old	Any loss of neurological function including altered or lost sensation, weakness of the limbs (either transiently or permanently) and alterations in bladder or bowel function
Vaginal trauma	Any history or other evidence of direct trauma to the vagina
Local infection	Local infection usually manifests as inflammation (pain, swelling and redness) confined to a particular site or area, with or without a collection of pus
Local inflammation	Local inflammation will involve pain, swelling and redness confined to a particular site or area

Discriminator dictionary

Discriminator	Definition
Abdominal pain	Any pain felt in the abdomen. Abdominal pain associated with back pain may indicate abdominal aortic aneurysm, while association with PV bleeding may indicate ectopic pregnancy or miscarriage
Abrupt onset	Onset within seconds or minutes. May cause waking from sleep
Acute chemical eye injury	Any substance splashed into or placed into the eye within the past 12 hours that caused stinging, burning or reduced vision should be assumed to have caused chemical injury
Acute complete loss of vision	Loss of vision in one or both eyes within the preceding 24 hours that has not returned to normal
Acute onset after injury	Onset of symptoms immediately within 24 hours of a physically traumatic event
Acutely avulsed tooth	A tooth that has been avulsed intact within the previous 24 hours
Acutely short of breath	Shortness of breath that comes on suddenly, or a sudden exacerbation of chronic shortness of breath
Age 25 years or less	Less than 25 years old
Airway compromise	An airway may be compromised either because it cannot be kept open or because the airway protective reflexes (that stop inhalation) have been lost. Failure to keep the airway open will result either in intermittent total obstruction or in partial obstruction. This will manifest itself as snoring or bubbling sounds during breathing
Altered conscious level	Not fully alert. Either responding to voice or pain only or unresponsive
Altered conscious level ***not*** wholly attributable to alcohol	A patient who is not fully alert, with a history of alcohol ingestion, and in whom there may be other causes of reduced conscious level
Altered conscious level wholly attributable to alcohol	A patient who is not fully alert, with a clear history of alcohol ingestion, and in whom there is no doubt that all other causes of reduced conscious level have been excluded
Altered facial sensation	Any alteration of sensation on the face
Aortic pain	The onset of symptoms is sudden and the leading symptom is severe abdominal or chest pain. The pain may be described as sharp, stabbing or ripping in character. Classically, aortic chest pain is felt around the sternum and then radiates to the shoulder blades; aortic abdominal pain is felt in the centre of the abdomen and radiates to the back. The pain may get better or even vanish and then recur elsewhere. Over time, pain may also be felt in the arms, neck, lower jaw, stomach or hips

Discriminator	Definition
Apparently hallucinating	Patients who are apparently hallucinating may appear distracted and may appear to react to stimuli (primarily visual and auditory) that are not apparent to anyone else
Atypical behaviour	Children who are behaving in a way that is not usual in the given situation. The carers will often volunteer this information. Such children are often referred to as fractious or 'out of sorts'
Auricular haematoma	A tense haematoma (usually post traumatic) in the outer ear
Black or redcurrant stools	Any blackness fulfils the criteria of black stool while a dark red stool, classically seen in intussusceptions, is redcurrant stool
Bleeding disorder	Congenital or acquired bleeding disorder
Cardiac pain	Classically, a severe dull 'gripping' or 'heavy' pain in the centre of the chest, radiating to the left arm or to the neck. May be associated with sweating and nausea. Some patients may be less likely to seek medical attention and treatment quickly, despite the warning signs
Chest injury	Any injury to the area below the clavicles and above the level of the lowest rib. Injury to the lower part of the chest can cause underlying damage to abdominal organs
Cold	If the skin feels cold the patient is clinically said to be cold. The temperature should be taken as soon as possible – a core temperature less than 35°C is cold
Colicky pain	Pain that comes and goes in waves. Renal colic tends to come and go over 20 minutes or so
Critical skin	A fracture or dislocation may leave fragments or ends of bone pressing so hard against the skin that the viability of the skin is threatened. The skin will be white and under tension
Current palpitations	A feeling of the heart racing (often described as a fluttering) that is still present
Currently fitting	Patients who are in the tonic or clonic stages of a grand mal convulsion, and patients currently experiencing partial fits
Deformity	This will always be subjective. Abnormal angulation or rotation is implied
Diplopia	Double vision that resolves when one eye is closed
Direct trauma to the back	This may be top to bottom (loading), for instance when people fall and land on their feet, bending (forwards, backwards or to the side) or twisting
Direct trauma to the neck	This may be top to bottom (loading), for instance when something falls on the head, bending (forwards, backwards or to the side) twisting or distracting such as hanging
Discharge	In the context of sexually acquired infection this is any discharge from the penis or abnormal discharge from the vagina
Discharged from mental health services within the last 15 days	Any patient who has been discharged from an active period of care under mental health services (in hospital or in the community) within the last 15 days
Disruptive	Disruptive behaviour is behaviour that affects the smooth running of the department. It may be threatening
Distal vascular compromise	There will be a combination of pallor, coldness, altered sensation and pain with or without absent pulses distal to the injury

Discriminator	Definition
Drooling	Saliva running from the mouth as a result of being unable to swallow
Dysuria	Pain or difficulty in passing urine. Pain is typically described as stinging or hot
Electrical injury	Any injury caused or possibly caused by an electric current. This includes AC and DC and both artificial and natural sources
Exhaustion	Exhausted patients appear to reduce the effort they make to breathe despite continuing respiratory insufficiency. This is pre-terminal
Exsanguinating haemorrhage	Haemorrhage which is occurring at such a rate that death will ensue unless bleeding is stopped
Externalisation of organs	Herniation or frank extrusion of internal organs
Extreme aggression or agitation requiring immediate restraint	Aggression and agitation of such a degree that immediate restraint is required to manage the risk of harm to self or others
Facial oedema	Diffuse swelling around the face, usually involving the lips
Facial swelling	Swelling around the face which may be localised or diffuse
Fails to react to parents	Failure to react in any way to a parent's face or voice. Abnormal reactions and apparent lack of recognition of a parent are also worrying signs
Floppy	Parents may describe their children as floppy. Tone is generally reduced – the most noticeable sign is often lolling of the head
Foreign body sensation	A sensation of something in the eye, often expressed as scraping or grittiness
Frank haematuria	Red discolouration of the urine caused by blood
Gross deformity	This will always be subjective. Gross and abnormal angulation or rotation is implied
Headache	Any pain around the head that is not related to a particular anatomical structure. Facial pain is not included
Heavy PV blood loss	PV loss is extremely difficult to assess. The presence of large clots or constant flow fulfils this criterion. The use of a large number of sanitary towels is suggestive of heavy loss
High blood pressure	A history of raised blood pressure or a raised blood pressure on examination
High lethality	Lethality is the potential of the substance taken to cause harm. Advice from a poisons centre may be required to establish the level of risk of serious illness or death. If in doubt, assume a high risk
High lethality chemical	Lethality is the potential of the chemical to cause harm. Advice may be required to establish the level of risk. If in doubt, assume a high risk
High lethality envenomation	Lethality is the potential of the envenomation to cause harm. Local knowledge may allow identification of the venomous creature, but advice may be required. If in doubt, assume a high risk
High risk of further self-harm	An initial view of the risk of harm to self can be formed by considering the patient's behaviour. Patients who are threatening to harm themselves and who are actively seeking the means to do so are at high risk
High risk of leaving before assessment	Active, credible threats to leave prior to assessment pose a high risk

Discriminator	Definition
High risk of self-harm	An initial view of the risk of harm to self can be formed by considering the patient's behaviour. Patients who are threatening to harm themselves and who are actively seeking the means to do so are at high risk
History of acutely vomiting blood	Frank haematemesis, vomiting of altered blood (coffee ground) or of blood mixed in the vomit within the past 24 hours
History of fitting	Any observed or reported fits that have occurred during the period of illness or following an episode of trauma
History of head injury	A history of a recent physically traumatic event involving the head. Usually this will be reported by the patient but if the patient has been unconscious this history should be sought from a reliable witness
History of overdose or poisoning	This information may come from others or may be deduced if medication is missing
History of recent foreign travel	Recent significant foreign travel (within 2 weeks)
History of trauma	A history of a recent physically traumatic event
History of unconsciousness	There may be a reliable witness who can state whether the patient was unconscious (and for how long). If not, a patient who is unable to remember the incident should be assumed to have been unconscious
Hot	If the skin feels hot the person is clinically said to be hot. The temperature should be taken as soon as possible – a temperature of 38.5°C and greater is hot
Hot baby	If the skin is hot, the child is clinically said to be hot. The temperature should be taken as soon as possible – a temperature of 38.5°C and greater is hot. A baby is a child less than 1 year old
Hot joint	Any warmth around a joint. Often accompanied by redness
Hyperglycaemia	Glucose greater than 17 mmol/l
Hyperglycaemia with ketosis	Glucose greater than 11 mmol/l with the presence of ketones. If unable to check for ketones, look for clinical signs of acidosis which may include deep rapid breathing, vomiting and confusion
Hypoglycaemia	Glucose less than 3 mmol/l
Immediate risk of leaving before assessment	Active, credible attempts to leave prior to assessment pose an immediate risk
Immediate risk to others	An initial view of the risk of harm to others can be judged by looking at posture (tense, clenched), speech (loud, using threatening words) and motor behaviour (restless, pacing, lunging at others). Immediate risk should be assumed if weapons and potential victims are available and no controls are already in place
Immediate risk to self	An initial view of the risk of harm to self can be formed by considering the patient's behaviour. Patients who are actively harming themselves and those who are threatening to harm themselves and who have the means to do so are at immediate risk
In active labour	A patient who is having regular and frequent painful contractions
Inadequate breathing	Patients who are failing to breathe well enough to maintain adequate oxygenation have inadequate breathing. There may be an increased work of breathing, signs of inadequate breathing or exhaustion
Inadequate history	If there is no clear and unequivocal history of acute alcohol ingestion, and if head injury, drug ingestion, underlying medical condition, etc. cannot be definitely excluded, then the history is inadequate

Discriminator	Definition
Inappropriate history	When the history (story) given does not explain the physical findings it is termed inappropriate. This is important as it is a marker of safeguarding concerns in both adults and children
Inconsolable by parents	Children whose crying or distress does not respond to attempts by their parents to comfort them
Increased work of breathing	Increased work of breathing is shown as increased respiratory rate, use of accessory muscles and grunting
Ingestion of a dangerous object	Ingestion of a dangerous or potentially dangerous foreign object, e.g. button battery, magnets or razor blades, which may be a potential threat to life
Inhalational injury	A history of being confined in a smoke-filled space is the most reliable indicator of smoke inhalation. Carbon deposits around the mouth and nose and hoarse voice may be present. History is also the most reliable way of diagnosing inhalation of chemicals – there will not necessarily be any signs
Jaundice	Neonatal jaundice
Known or likely immunosuppression	Any patient who is known or likely to be immunosuppressed including those on immunosuppressive drugs (including long-term steroids)
Likely to require admission under mental health legislation	Patients with significant psychiatric symptoms who are likely to require admission under mental health legislation
Local infection	Local infection usually manifests as inflammation (pain, swelling and redness) confined to a particular site or area, with or without a collection of pus
Local inflammation	Local inflammation will involve pain, swelling and redness confined to a particular site or area
Low PEFR	The PEFR predicted after consideration of the age and sex of the patient. Some patients may know their 'best' PEFR and this may be used. If the ratio of measured to predicted is less than 50% then this criterion is fulfilled
Low SpO_2	This is a saturation of less than 95% on air. The variation in risk according to skin colour necessitates the integration of pulse oximetry with other clinical and patient-reported data
Lower abdominal pain	Any pain felt in the lower abdomen; in association with PV bleeding may indicate ectopic pregnancy or miscarriage
Marked distress	Patients who are markedly physically or emotionally upset
Massive haemoptysis	Coughing up large amounts of fresh or clotted blood. Not to be confused with streaks of blood in saliva
Moderate aggression or agitation	Agitation or aggression that can usually be managed by verbal de-escalation without physical restraint
Moderate lethality	Lethality is the potential of the substance taken to cause serious illness or death. Advice from a poisons centre may be required to establish the level of risk to the patient
Moderate lethality chemical	Lethality is the potential of the chemical to cause harm. Advice may be required to establish the level of risk. If in doubt, assume a high risk

Discriminator	Definition
Moderate lethality envenomation	Lethality is the potential of the envenomation to cause harm. Local knowledge may allow identification of the venomous creature, but advice may be required
Moderate pain	Pain that is bearable but intense
Moderate pain or itch	Pain or itch that is bearable but intense
Moderate risk of further self-harm	An initial view of the risk of harm to self can be formed by considering the patient's behaviour. Patients without a significant history of self-harm, who are not actively trying to harm themselves, but who profess the desire to harm themselves are at moderate risk
Moderate risk of harm to others	An initial view of the risk of harm to others can be judged by looking at posture (tense, clenched), speech (loud, using threatening words) and motor behaviour (restless, pacing, lunging at others). Moderate risk should be assumed if there is any indication of potential harm to others
Moderate risk of leaving before assessment	Threats to leave without any attempts to do so pose a moderate risk
Moderate risk of self-harm	An initial view of the risk of harm to self can be formed by considering the patient's behaviour. Patients without a significant history of self-harm, who are not actively trying to harm themselves, but who profess the desire to harm themselves are at moderate risk
New abnormal pulse	A bradycardia (less than 60 beats per minute in adults), a tachycardia (more than 100 beats per minute in adults) or an irregular rhythm. Age-appropriate definitions of bradycardia and tachycardia should be used in children
New confusion	Patients with new onset confusion
New continuous vertigo	New sensation of dizziness or vertigo which is continuous, and which has started within the previous 24 hours
New neurological deficit less than 24 hours old	Any loss of neurological function that has come on within the previous 24 hours. This might include altered or lost sensation, weakness of the limbs (either transiently or permanently) and alterations in bladder or bowel function
New neurological deficit more than 24 hours old	Any loss of neurological function including altered or lost sensation, weakness of the limbs (either transiently or permanently) and alterations in bladder or bowel function
New onset of significant mental health symptoms	Any new mental health symptoms not already taken into account
New symptoms of psychosis	Active new symptoms of psychosis with no insight such as hallucinations, delusions and/or paranoia
No improvement with own asthma medications	This history should be available from the patient. A failure to improve with bronchodilator therapy given by the GP or paramedic is equally significant
Non-blanching rash	A rash that does not blanch (go white) when pressure is applied to it. Often tested using a glass tumbler to apply pressure as any colour change can be observed through the bottom of the tumbler
Not distractible	Children who are distressed by pain or other things who cannot be distracted by conversation or play
Not feeding	Children who will not take any solid or liquid (as appropriate) by mouth. Children who will take the food but always vomit afterwards may also fulfil this criterion

Discriminator	Definition
Not passing urine	Failure to produce and pass urine. This may be difficult to judge in children (and the elderly) and reference to the number of nappies or pads used may be useful
Oedema of the tongue	Swelling of the tongue of any degree
Open fracture	All wounds in the vicinity of a fracture should be regarded with suspicion. If there is any possibility of communication between the wound and the fracture then the fracture should be assumed to be open
Pain on joint movement	This can be pain on either active (patient) movement or passive (examiner) movement
Passing fresh or altered blood PR	In active massive GI bleeding, dark red blood will be passed PR. As GI transit time increases this becomes darker, eventually becoming melaena
Penetrating eye injury	A recent physically traumatic event involving penetration of the globe
Persistent vomiting	Vomiting that is continuous or that occurs without any respite between episodes
Pleuritic pain	A sharp, localised pain in the chest that worsens on breathing, coughing or sneezing
Possible sepsis	Suspected sepsis in patients who present with altered mental state, low blood pressure (systolic less than 100 mmHg) or raised respiratory rate (rate more than 22 breaths per minute) when using the qSOFA tool for assessment. Other sepsis screening tools may be used instead of qSOFA, and the relevant sepsis markers applied. In children, age-specific physiological tools should be used to determine if possibly septic
Possibly pregnant	Any patient whose normal menstruation has failed to occur is possibly pregnant and any patient, of child-bearing age, who is having unprotected sex should be considered to be potentially pregnant
Presenting foetal parts	Crowning or presentation of any other foetal part in the vagina
Priapism	Sustained penile erection
Productive cough	A cough that is productive of phlegm, whatever the colour
Prolapsed umbilical cord	Prolapse of any part of the umbilical cord through the cervix
Prolonged or uninterrupted crying	A child who has cried continuously for 2 hours or more
Purpura	A rash on any part of the body that is caused by small haemorrhages under the skin. A purpuric rash does not blanch (go white) when pressure is applied to it
PV blood loss	Any loss of blood PV
PV blood loss and 20 weeks pregnant or more	Any loss of blood PV in a patient known to be beyond the 20th week of pregnancy
Rapid onset	Onset within the preceding 12 hours
Recent dizziness or vertigo	An acute feeling of spinning or dizziness, possibly accompanied by nausea and vomiting
Recent hearing loss	Loss of hearing in one or both ears within the previous week
Recent injury	An injury occurring within the last week

Discriminator	Definition
Recent mild pain	Any pain that has occurred within the past 7 days
Recent mild pain or itch	Any pain or itch that has occurred within the past 7 days
Recent problem	A problem arising in the last week
Recent reduced visual acuity	Any reduction in corrected visual acuity within the past 7 days
Recent signs of mild pain	Young children and babies in pain cannot complain. They will usually cry occasionally and may act atypically
Recently given birth	A patient who has given birth within the past 3 months
Red eye	Any redness to the eye. A red eye may be painful or painless and may be complete or partial
Reduced foetal movements >20 weeks	Absent or reduced foetal movements during the previous 12 hours in a patient known to be beyond the 20th week of pregnancy
Responds to voice or pain only	Responds to painful stimuli, which could include standard peripheral stimuli – a pen or pencil is used to apply pressure to the finger or nail bed. The stimulus should not be applied to the toes since a spinal reflex may cause flexion even in brain death. Central stimuli such as trapezius squeeze or supraorbital ridge pressure can be used but clinicians should be aware reflex grimacing may occur It is not necessary to shout the patient's name. Children may fail to respond because they are afraid
Retention of urine	Inability to pass urine per urethra associated with an enlarged bladder. This condition is usually very painful unless there is altered sensation
Risk of continued contamination	If chemical exposure is likely to continue (usually due to lack of adequate decontamination) then this discriminator applies. Risks to healthcare workers must not be forgotten if this situation occurs
Safeguarding concerns	Any concerns for the welfare of the patient that arise from their vulnerability
Scalp haematoma	A raised bruised area to the scalp (bruises below the hair line at the front are to the forehead)
Scrotal cellulitis	Redness and swelling around the scrotum
Scrotal gangrene	Dead, blackened skin around the scrotum and groin. Early gangrene may not be black but may appear like a full-thickness burn with or without flaking
Scrotal trauma	Any recent physically traumatic event involving the scrotum
Self-harmed without other psychiatric disease	Patients who have harmed themselves (for the first or subsequent time) who do not have a mental health diagnosis
Severe aggression or agitation that may require restraint	Aggression and agitation of such a degree that restraint may be required at short notice to manage the risk of harm to self or others
Severe pain	Pain that is unbearable – often described as the worst ever
Severe pain or itch	Pain or itch that is unbearable – often described as the worst ever
Severe tachypnoea	A child less than 1 year with a respiratory rate of 55 breaths per minute or above ***OR*** a child 1 year or above with a respiratory rate of 45 breaths per minute or above
Severe tachypnoea in children	A child less than 1 year with a respiratory rate of 55 breaths per minute or above ***OR*** a child 1 year or above with a respiratory rate of 45 breaths per minute or above

Discriminator	Definition
Shock	Shock is inadequate delivery of oxygen to the tissues. The classic signs include sweating, pallor, tachycardia, hypotension and reduced conscious level
Shoulder tip pain	Pain felt in the tip of the shoulder. This often indicates diaphragmatic irritation
Significant cardiac history	A known recurrent dysrhythmia that has life-threatening effects is significant, as is a known cardiac condition which may deteriorate rapidly
Significant haematological or metabolic history	A patient with a significant haematological condition or a congenital metabolic disorder that is known to deteriorate rapidly
Significant history of allergy	A known sensitivity with severe reaction (e.g. to nuts or bee sting) is significant
Significant history of GI bleed	Any history of massive GI bleeding or of any GI bleeding associated with oesophageal varices
Significant mechanism of injury	Penetrating injuries (stab or gunshot) and injuries with high energy transfer. In the frail/elderly, low energy transfer such as a fall from standing may be significant
Significant medical history	Any pre-existing medical condition requiring continual medication or other care
Significant psychiatric history	A history of a major psychiatric illness or event
Significant respiratory history	A history of previous life-threatening episodes of a respiratory condition (e.g. COPD) is significant, as is brittle asthma
Signs of dehydration	These include dry tongue, sunken eyes, decreased skin turgor and, in small babies, a sunken anterior fontanelle. Usually associated with a low urine output
Signs of meningism	Classically, a stiff neck together with headache and photophobia
Signs of moderate pain	Young children and babies in moderate pain cannot complain. They will usually cry intermittently and are often intermittently consolable
Signs of severe pain	Young children and babies in severe pain cannot complain. They will usually cry out continuously and inconsolably and be tachycardic. They may well exhibit signs such as pallor and sweating
Smoke exposure	Smoke inhalation should be assumed if the patient has been confined in a smoke-filled space. Physical signs such as oral or nasal soot are less reliable but significant if present
Special risk of infection	Known exposure to a dangerous pathogen, or travel to an area with an identified, current, serious infectious risk
Stridor	This may be an inspiratory or expiratory noise, or both. Stridor is heard best on breathing with the mouth open.
Subcutaneous gas	Gas under the skin can be detected by feeling for a 'crackling' on touch. There may be gas bubbles and a line of demarcation
Swelling	An abnormal increase in size
Tachycardia in children	A child less than 1 year with a heart rate of 160 bpm or above ***OR*** a child 1 year or above with a heart rate of 140 bpm or above

Discriminator	Definition
Tachypnoea	A child less than 1 year with a respiratory rate of 45 breaths per minute or above ***OR*** a child 1 year or above with a respiratory rate of 35 breaths per minute or above
Tachypnoea in children	A child less than 1 year with a respiratory rate of 45 breaths per minute or above ***OR*** a child 1 year or above with a respiratory rate of 35 breaths per minute or above
Temporal scalp tenderness	Tenderness on palpation over the temporal area (especially over the artery)
Testicular pain	Pain in the testicles
Threats of violence or high risk of harm to others	An initial view of the risk of harm to others can be judged by looking at posture (tense, clenched), speech (loud, using threatening words) and motor behaviour (restless, pacing, lunging at others). High risk should be assumed if potential victims are available and inadequate controls are in place
Unable to feed	This is usually reported by the parents. Children who will not take any solid or liquid (as appropriate) by mouth
Unable to talk in sentences	Patients who are so breathless that they cannot complete relatively short sentences in one breath
Unable to walk	It is important to try and distinguish between patients who have pain and difficulty walking and those who cannot walk. Only the latter can be said to be unable to walk
Uncontrollable major haemorrhage	A haemorrhage that is not rapidly controlled by the application of sustained direct pressure and in which blood continues to flow heavily or soak through large dressings quickly
Uncontrollable minor haemorrhage	A haemorrhage that is not rapidly controlled by the application of sustained direct pressure and in which blood continues to flow slightly or ooze
Unresponsive	A child who fails to respond to either verbal or painful stimuli
Unresponsive child	A child who fails to respond to either verbal or painful stimuli
Vaginal trauma	Any history or other evidence of direct trauma to the vagina
Vascular compromise	There will be a combination of pallor, coldness, altered sensation and pain with or without absent pulses distal to the injury
Vertigo	An acute feeling of spinning or dizziness, possibly accompanied by nausea and vomiting
Very hot	If the skin feels very hot the patient is clinically said to be very hot. The temperature should be taken as soon as possible – a temperature of 41°C or greater is very hot
Very low PEFR	The PEFR predicted after consideration of the age and sex of the patient. Some patients may know their 'best' PEFR and this may be used. If the ratio of measured to predicted is less than 33% then this criterion is fulfilled
Very low SpO_2	This is a saturation of less than 95% on O_2 therapy or less than 92% on air. The variation in risk according to skin colour necessitates the integration of pulse oximetry with other clinical and patient-reported data

Discriminator	Definition
Visible abdominal mass	A mass in the abdomen that is visible to the naked eye
Vomiting	Any emesis
Vomiting blood	Vomited blood may be fresh (bright or dark red) or coffee ground in appearance
Warm	If the skin feels warm the patient is clinically said to be warm. The temperature should be taken as soon as possible – a temperature greater than 37.5°C is warm
Warm newborn	If the skin feels warm the patient is clinically said to be warm. The temperature should be taken as soon as possible – a child of 28 days or under with a temperature of 37.5–38.4°C is warm
Wheeze	This can be audible wheeze or a feeling of wheeze. Very severe airway obstruction is silent (no air can move)
Widespread discharge or blistering	Any discharging or blistering eruption covering more than 10% of the body surface area
Widespread rash or blistering	Any rash or blistering eruption covering more than 10% of the body surface area

Further reading

Mackway-Jones AJ, Mackway-Jones KC (2020) An Expert Delphi study to derive a tool for mental health triage in emergency departments. *Emerg Med J* 37: 738–743.

Mackway-Jones A, Hornby R, Mackway-Jones K (2023) Making more nurses, one minute at a time: an efficiency and quality improvement project in emergency triage. *Emerg Nurse* DOI: 10.7748/en.2023.e2127.

van Veen M, Steyerberg EW, Van't Klooster M, Ruige M, van Meurs AHJ, van der Lei J, Henriëtte A, Moll HA (2012) The Manchester Triage System: improvements for paediatric emergency care. *Emerg Med J* 29: 654–659.

Zachariasse JM, Maconochie IK, Nijman RG, Greber-Platzer S, Smit FJ, Nieboer D, van der Lei J, Alves CF, Moll H (2021) Improving the prioritization of children at the emergency department: updating the Manchester Triage System using vital signs. *PLOS One* 16(2): e0246324.

Abbreviations

A&E	Accident and emergency
ABC	Airway, breathing and circulation
ABCD	Airway, breathing, circulation and disability
AC	Alternating current
ALSG	Advanced Life Support Group
COPD	Chronic obstructive pulmonary disease
DC	Direct current
ECG	Electrocardiography
ED	Emergency department
FLACC	Faces, legs, activity, cry and consolability
GCS	Glasgow coma score
GI	Gastrointestinal
GP	General practitioner
GPT	Grupo Português de Triagem
IRGs	International Reference Groups
LOC	Loss of consciousness
Ma	Majors area
MAU	Medical assessment unit
Mi	Minors area
MTS	Manchester Triage System
PAINAD	Pain assessment in advanced dementia
PAU	Paediatric assessment unit
PC	Primary care
PEFR	Peak expiratory flow rate
PGDs	Patient group directions
PPM	Presentation–priority matrix
PR	Per rectum
PV	Per vaginum
qSOFA	Quick sequential organ failure assessment
RR	Respiratory rate
SAU	Surgical assessment unit
SC	Self-care
SDEC	Same day emergency care
SHC	Sexual health clinic
TCM	Time critical medications
UK	United Kingdom
UTC	Urgent treatment centre

Index

Page references for the presentation flowcharts and chart notes are given in bold type.